SMART FITTness
Focused Time-Efficient Conditioning

By David Jed Squires,

B.A. Physical Education/Exercise Science

Masters of Arts in Teaching

SMART FITTness PUBLICATIONS

SMART FITTness
Focused Time-Efficient Conditioning

Copyright 2007© David Jed Squires
Revised 2010, 2019
SMART FITTness PUBLICATIONS
All rights reserved.

ISBN #9781702590082

Line Drawings
Charlyn Bokum
cjbokum@gmail.com

To order additional copies contact me at:
coachdavid@smartfittness.com

ACKNOWLEDGEMENTS
GREAT **BIG**
THANK YOU'S

First, I give praise to the Lord for without His presence through the Holy Spirit I would not have been able to write this book. There were times when doubt crept in and I wondered if this was something I could really do. I put the book aside for months at a time, but the Holy Spirit continued to work on both the material and me. I had started a worthwhile endeavor and it was important that I complete it.

As I wrote and edited this book, one of its principle themes served as a constant reminder:

"All things are possible to him who believes." Mark 9:23 NASB

To my wife whose tough love provided additional stimulus to get it done. Thank you, my love, for your continued support and challenging me to be the best that I can be.

To my parents and big brother who taught me the value of working hard and doing my best. Thank you for encouraging me in whatever path I chose and providing love and support along the way.

So many people over the years have provided feedback, both in the form of encouragement and suggestions that I fear missing someone. If you are one of those people and your name does not appear here, please forgive me. Charge it to my head, not to my heart as I greatly appreciate everyone who contributed.

Special thanks go out to Glenn Wilkensen. Glenn gave one of my early drafts a thorough review and provided many useful suggestions. Others who provided valuable feedback include: Jason Barbacovi, Dan Clark, Darren Siegel, Richard Isral, Paul Clark, Jim Muldoon, Todd Bergmann, and Laura Partlow.

CONTENTS

PREFACE
KNOW THE MESSENGER FIRST

When I first started to write this book, I decided it was important for you to know a bit about me personally, and in particular how I developed my approach to health and fitness. I knew instinctively that it was important to share my story, however I did not give it much thought beyond that. That was until recently, when I was reminded of an important lesson I had learned early on in life: "People don't care how much I know, until they know how much I care."

I understand there are a lot of *experts* offering information about health and fitness. So why should you listen to me? Well, I am going to answer that very important question in the Forward, *My Story,* and the Introduction, *Why I Wrote This Book*. So, before you hear my message, go ahead and get to know me, the messenger, first.

FORWARD

MY STORY

<u>**Passion for Sport and Achievement**</u>

Many people have influenced my life and, in particular, my decision to pursue a career in fitness. It started at the age of eight in a local city Track & Field program. My first coach was a man named Barry Savage, whose unforgettable intensity and passion for life was truly inspirational.

The first day of practice he told us that we could count on him being there every day. He would never miss a day he said, "Because I never get sick." He didn't believe in getting sick and, during the time that I knew him, he never was. It was an early lesson on how thoughts directly affect our body's condition.

As a fitness professional for many years, I have continued to learn from a great number of teachers and coaches. At every level, primary school through college, these dedicated professionals have influenced my approach not only to health and wellness, but also to life. My passion and drive, due in large part to my mentors, has led me to compete in a wide variety of sports, over 20 at last count. Some of my favorites include: basketball, football, snow skiing, water skiing, rowing, power lifting, triathlons, tennis and squash. I have encountered many coaches over the years and I learned something from each and every one of them.

One coach in particular, Richard Yonk, made a strong impact in my life. In addition to being my offensive line coach in high school football, he was also the teacher of my *Weight Training and Conditioning* class. It was during this time that I learned the power of goal setting and visualization.

You see, there were these powerful, motivating **records** posted in the locker room—records for everything from 40-yard dash time to bench press and bar dips. It wasn't long before I had my sights set on a few of them and having done so began working out like never before.

One of my brother's friends happened to set the bench press record (1 rep at 340 pounds) during his senior, which was my sophomore, year. I remember like it was yesterday, vowing to break that record before I graduated.

Over the course of the next three years I worked toward this, and a few other fitness related goals. I enrolled in *Weight Training and Conditioning* as my first period class for the next three years in high school. As I worked out each day, increasing my strength and improving my technique, I knew that before I graduated, I would hold the bench press record. There was never a moment that I considered *if* I would break the record. My preparation was so complete that **I knew** I would do it. I saw it first in my mind's eye, and my body followed.

Just a few weeks before the end of my senior year, I broke the school bench press record (1 rep at 355 lbs.). I also broke the jump rope and arm curl records. At the time I did not realize how goal setting provided the stimulus to drive me toward these achievements. I know now that without having specific records (goals) to aim for, together with the power of visualization as a stimulus it would not have happened.

Finding My Way

Following high school, I decided to study Physical Education in order to become a teacher and coach. I wanted to help others, the way my mentors had helped me. Before attending university, I went to Community College to play football and improve my study habits. Moving to a school outside my home town meant adjusting to many different things at once: independence, college, and athletics at a higher level.

This proved to be a difficult time in my life: I was not prepared for the changes that took place. I neglected to apply the lessons of goal setting and visualization I learned early in life. They had not become a habit and without a clear goal my performance, both academic and athletic, declined.

My football playing days ended as it became clear I did not have the size or speed to compete at the next level. Since the age of eight I had been active in sports, and now for the first time in my life, I didn't know what to do next. With no new sport or activity in mind, the motivation to workout was gone. I started to get fat and out of shape; I needed something to get me going again.

Later that year, a friend of mine told me about an upcoming bodybuilding contest and encouraged me to enter. He invited me to the gym he trained at, and introduced me to the owner. Soon I was pumping iron again, this time purely for aesthetic reasons. In addition to my workouts, I began to learn more about proper nutrition and improved my eating habits.

Like most of us, I had grown up on the traditional meat and potatoes diet and loved fast food. For many years I considered junk food to be one of the four food groups. I soon found out that much of the food I was used to eating, was now unacceptable fair. With guidance from some friends at the gym, I began eating a whole foods based diet consisting of lean meats, fish, eggs, whole grains, fruits and vegetables. As before, mentors showed me the way.

Once again, I had a goal. The contest date was set, and I had to be ready to present my body for the judges and everyone in the audience to see. And if you haven't seen what a posing suit looks like, you should know there is not much left to the imagination. I remember mine arrived in the mail in a *small* envelope. I pulled my burgundy suit out of the package and tried it on. It was obvious I still had a way to go before I could wear it proudly.

Over the next 3½ months I worked out six days per week, two hours each day. By combining rigorous training and a natural diet I went from a fat, out of shape 199 pounds, to a lean, muscular 175. I did this without the use of steroids, and in fact at no time in my life have I ever used performance-enhancing drugs.

Training for this contest was one of the most demanding things I have ever done. Although I didn't win (I placed 7th out of 18 in my weight class), the experience proved valuable as it reinforced the idea that I could do anything that I set my mind to. The experience also raised my interest in Fitness, leading me to change my course of study to Exercise and Sports Science.

University – The Science of Exercise

The following year, I transferred to university to begin my degree work in physical education. One of the first courses I took was *Anatomy and Physiology*. While studying bones, muscles, and the many body systems my fascination for the human body continued to grow.

During these early university years something else made me particularly interested in how the body works, *rowing*. Having little knowledge about the sport I attended an informational meeting. Many of the seasoned rowers spoke at the meeting, and they all talked about the commitment and hard work that would be expected of anyone who turned out. Sacrifices would have to be made and that you would either love it or hate it. I found a real camaraderie among the crew and decided that would be my next challenge.

Before I knew it, I was waking up before dawn for practice. The best time of the day to get smooth water was in the morning, something I had learned years earlier waking up early to go water skiing. But what I didn't know was how physically challenging rowing would be.

Every day before practice, my teammates and I would go on what our coach optimistically called a *warm-up* run. Still half asleep and feeling the morning chill we would work our way along the lake shore. Since the run was typically a few miles long, most of us first year rowers were so tired from this warm-up the last thing we wanted to do was row. After a couple of weeks however, our bodies adapted to these morning jaunts, and we became primed and ready to row.

Rowing is a very technical sport. The boats (crew shells) used for rowing are very narrow, and the seats are on a slide. Your feet are strapped into shoes (stretchers) so that you can generate leverage with your whole body (legs, torso and arms). Rowing in both four and eight-person boats each of our movements had to be performed together as if moving as one. To achieve this objective, we practiced proper stroke mechanics, often twice a day. As we improved our technique and timing, we began to move as one.

As our technique improved, we picked up the pace. The amount of power we generated together was tremendous, and our boat really started to move. For conditioning purposes, we worked on longer distances to improve endurance and shorter ones to increase our power.

It was during, or rather after completing one of our shorter sprints where I began to notice the effects of our training. During practice one day, as we were working our way through a particularly difficult workout, I found something had changed. At the end of each segment my teammates and I were always out of breath. But on this day, although we were still winded, the amount of time needed to recover was much shorter. We went from gasping for air one minute to breathing normally just a short time later. Our bodies had once again adapted to the demands placed on them, just like with our warm-up run.

As I considered the many physical changes my body had gone through over the years, my knowledge and passion for this amazing machine we call the *human body* continued to grow. I didn't know it at the time, but my passion for fitness would take me to places I never dreamed and open up a world of possibilities.

Sharing My Passion

Over the next few years, I continued to study Exercise Science: Biomechanics (exercise's relationship to physics), Kinesiology (the study of movement), Exercise Physiology (the body's response to increased physical demands) and other pertinent courses. In addition to my course work, a practicum was organized at a clinic nearby the university. Most of the people coming to the clinic were either recovering from an orthopedic injury such as a torn knee ligament or an illness such as heart disease. It wasn't long before I knew this was not the environment for me. I wanted to focus on the prevention of such conditions, not treating them.

My next practicum was arranged at the local Athletic Club, which I found to be more suited to my interests. Following a few days of observation at the club, I arranged for my internship to be done there. It was time to share my knowledge and passion for fitness with others.

I remember being a bit nervous at first, as I had never instructed someone I didn't already know. Many of the questions in the *Risk Assessment Survey* were quite personal and required people to open up a great deal. I was surprised to find most people eager to tell me their stories.

Some of our members had specific goals they wanted to achieve with regard to their fitness level, while others did not. Yet again I was shown the power of goal setting, as the people that set written goals and kept them foremost in their minds made the most dramatic changes in their fitness levels.

Following my internship in 1985 I was hired on part-time as a *Fitness Consultant.* Since then, apart from a few breaks for extended travel and a job with a Seattle based dot.com venture (that went dot gone), I have continued working in the Fitness Industry.

During my career I have never stopped learning. I believe continuing education is vitally important because if you are not improving, you are going backwards. I have been fortunate to learn from a number of excellent fitness professionals: Randy Huntington, Tom Purvis and Neal Wolkodoff to name just a few. Lessons learned from these experts have taught me a great deal; however, the knowledge I have gained working with people like you has been of even greater value. I am forever grateful to all of you, as without your efforts and feedback I would not be where I am today.

Life Changing Experience

During the summer of 1997 I had decided to move to a bigger city. I had been living and working in smaller towns the six years following my college graduation. The town I spent most of my time was a population of about 65,000 people, and at this time I felt I needed to enter a larger market to further my career. I had no idea how much larger a market I was about to experience.

After the move I began to network with some Fitness Professionals in the area. A week later, standing in the kitchen of my new home, I received a life changing phone call. One of my contacts referred me to a group of clubs: *Clark Hatch Fitness Centers*. It turns out they were looking for a Club Manager at the time, but there was a bit of a twist. *Clark Hatch Fitness Centers* operates in Asia Pacific.

Clark Hatch is an American who was first in Asia during the Korean War. Following the war, he decided to remain in Asia and opened his first fitness center in Tokyo, Japan in 1965. Later, as he traveled about Asia, he found many of the hotels were lacking quality fitness centers. There was a need for professional consulting and management services within the major hotels, and he began to fill that need. Today, *Clark Hatch* still has many clubs throughout Asia Pacific, most of which are within 5-star hotels.

So here I was, just getting settled into my new home, and I was presented with the opportunity to move to Asia. The company was to pay my air ticket to Honolulu, Hawaii, and then on to Tokyo, Japan or Shanghai, China.

With a sense of adventure and interest in learning about another culture up-close, I decided to accept the offer. A few weeks later, I was on a plane to Honolulu to meet Mr. Hatch himself and begin my training. I spent three weeks in Honolulu for orientation and taking in the sites until the Shanghai Hilton was confirmed as my destination.

Following a brief trip through Hong Kong as part of my Visa processing, I arrived in Shanghai. I will never forget my first trip from the airport to the hotel, as it was unlike anything I had ever seen before. A sea of people, mostly on bicycles, moved about in a steady, unending stream. It is one thing to hear about 15 million people living in a city, yet another to experience it.

Over the course of the next few years, I learned about Chinese people and their long-held understanding of the importance of health. One indication was held within a greeting used for many years. The word for body's health is "*shen ti*" and there was a time when it was customary to greet a person with: "shen ti hao ma?" Which means, "How's your body's health?"

This greeting is not so common today; in fact, just like in other developed countries many people within China's larger cities are sacrificing their health in the quest to make more money. Although you still can find a large number of people throughout the city practicing tai chi, jogging, dancing or performing some other form of movement, the numbers are dwindling. In addition, the majority of people you see committed to these activities are senior citizens. Although it is great to see the older generation staying active, it is sad to see the rest of the population going the way of the "modern world."

Young people within China today have taken to junk food and computer games, and their parents have focused their energy on creating more of everything, except wellness that is. And while nobody can argue the importance of making money, no matter how much money you make, it is of little value if you are not physically able to enjoy it.

A Fruitful Search

One day while searching online for fitness information I discovered a man named Matt Furey. As a lifetime student I am forever seeking new information, and in this case my search proved particularly fruitful. There is a great deal of information about health and fitness online, some of which is questionable at best. Matt, however, is the real deal. While reading his story, I became truly inspired as I identified with many of Matt's experiences and share much of his fitness philosophy.

Matt is an advocate of body weight exercises; a form of which I have always felt deserved more attention. Consider that, pound for pound, the strongest, most powerful, yet incredibly flexible athletes on this earth are ones that condition themselves through body weight exercises. Gymnasts, wrestlers, dancers, and martial artists all leave little doubt this type of exercise works.

Although I had incorporated calisthenics into both my client's routines, and mine they were never the foundation of the program. Until discovering Matt's program, I had used body weight exercises as an alternative to weight training when weights were inaccessible, or for a change of pace in my workouts.

I remember one particular occasion, working out in a club that I also worked as a *Personal Trainer*. The facility was well equipped with both strength training and cardiovascular machines valued at well over $100,000. Yet here I was, down on the floor doing push-ups. Mike, one of our regular members looked over at me like I was crazy and asked, "Why are doing push-ups when you could be benching?" My answer at the time was, "just for some variety." Looking back, I believe intuitively I knew that push-ups provided a better overall workout than the bench press. Possibly, the only reason I lifted weights all those years was due to influence from outside sources telling me lifting weights was the *only* or *best* way to improve my strength.

Although I still believe in lifting weights, I no longer believe it is the best way to condition our muscles. Since altering my workouts to include a variety of body weight exercises as the foundation of my program, my overall condition has never been better. I am strong, flexible, and have excellent endurance. I can participate in virtually any activity I choose, without undue fatigue.

During my career I have written various articles on Health and Fitness, published primarily in newsletters and regional magazines. I have considered writing a book several times. I just never set a goal to do so. Like most dreams the idea was just floating around in my mind with no real impetus to "get it together." Now, after years of formal education and valuable, real-life experience, I am ready to share my methods with you. It is my sincere desire that the information contained within this book will change your life. I know writing it has changed mine.

Update

Since writing the first edition of this book a lot has happened both personally and professionally. My wife Cherry gave birth to our son Joshua in 2007. He has provided great joy in our lives and provided us with the ultimate challenge of being a parent.

Career wise, after serving as Director of Eagle Gate College's Personal Fitness Training program for over five years, I returned to school to earn a Master's in Teaching from Westminster College. Earning a Master's in Teaching at Westminster College was a great experience, reinforcing many concepts in this book. There were times when the workload felt overwhelming, and I had to remind myself to just focus on each project individually. Doing this allowed be to perform at my best and complete the program with high marks.

Following graduation, I have been teaching at the secondary level in Health and Physical Education. Sharing my passion for my subject matter with my students has been a rewarding experience. During this time, I have also continued coaching, utilizing many of the principles taught in this book.

My experiences as a Performance Coach have reinforced the value of goal setting, a natural whole foods diet, and an activity program based on body weight exercises.

The journey continues, and I cannot wait to experience the challenges that lie ahead in the years to come.

INTRODUCTION
WHY I WROTE THIS BOOK

One thing we are not lacking today is information about health and fitness. It seems a new book comes out every day with some great *new* program that is guaranteed to help you lose weight and shape up. And while some of the information provided is of value, much of it is questionable at best.

Few programs provide the essential components necessary for you to improve your health and fitness. They lack the vital mental conditioning so important in lifestyle change and the activity programs are often too difficult for people to fit into their busy lives.

As an active professional and family man I understand the need for a focused, time-efficient program that works. Our lives have become increasingly busy; between work pressures and family responsibilities it seems there is never enough time in the day. Within this stress filled, hurry up world our health is often neglected. This is a big mistake for a number of reasons, most of all because...

Without your health, nothing else matters.

Take some time and think about that for a minute. How much can you accomplish if you are lying in a hospital bed recovering from a heart attack? How much joy is there in life if you are suffering from cancer? How well can you move around if you suffer a stroke or experience frequent back pain?

The conditions listed above are more prevalent today than ever before, and it is not by accident. Our modern lifestyle is responsible for this fact. We have become increasingly inactive, and the type and quantity of foods we eat are often less than ideal. Many people continue down this path thinking they are somehow different, *invincible*. You may think, "It just couldn't happen to me." Well guess what: it has happened to hundreds of millions of people just like you, so how are you any different?

In fact, these diseases and a variety of other ailments have become so common, it seems everyone knows at least one person who has, or currently is, suffering from ill health. Unfortunately, I have witnessed this within my own family. My mother died of colon cancer in her early forties, my stepmother also died of cancer recently at age 84, and my father has battled various health issues as well.

Thankfully, much of this is disease preventable. A few simple lifestyle changes will make all the difference in the world with regard to your health. While simple certainly does not mean easy, with a desire for change and the knowledge to do so anything is possible.

This book provides the tools necessary to change your lifestyle and regain your most important asset, your health. No matter what your age or present condition, there is hope for a more energetic, productive you.

Before we get into some of the specifics of the program, let's first consider an important correlation between...

Health and Fitness

There is some debate with regard to the difference between health and fitness. Many people still consider health to be defined by an absence of illness. Their logic tells them, "If I am not currently sick, then I must be well." Whether you believe this to be true or not depends on your definition of health. The WHO (World Health Organization) now defines health as: "*A state of complete physical, mental, and social well-being and **not merely** the absence of disease or infirmity.*" When it comes to defining *fitness,* there are various descriptions used, most of which are too vague. General fitness, as defined by *thefreedictionary.com,* is: *good physical condition, being in shape or condition*. But what is "*good physical condition.*" What is considered good to one person may not be acceptable to another.

The most common definition of fitness used by health professional's targets one particular component of fitness, cardiovascular. The volume of oxygen you can consume while exercising at maximum intensity (VO2 Max as it is often referred) is a common indicator. But what about the other components of fitness like muscular strength, flexibility, balance, and body composition? Are they any less important? What if someone has a high VO2 Max but still lacks the strength necessary to pick up a box of books and carry it up a couple flights of stairs. Can they really be considered physically fit?

A general, yet more practical definition of fitness is *having enough energy to complete your daily tasks while still having energy left over for leisure time pursuits or to meet any emergency demands*. This definition does have its limits though, as your desired fitness level would vary based on your daily energy requirements and leisure pursuits. Clearly, if you have a desk job and your leisure pursuit is a stroll around the park, the fitness level required is much different than for someone who works physically hard and/or wants to play competitive tennis.

Although you will find the words Health and Fitness used somewhat interchangeably within this book, in my mind, to be truly healthy one must maintain at least a moderate level of fitness. This is confirmed by numerous studies, including recent research published by the British Journal of Sports Medicine and the Journal of the American Medical Association. Both studies confirm an active lifestyle that leads to greater levels of fitness have a meaningful impact on health and longevity.

Fitness with a Purpose

While delaying mortality is well and good, I do not know many people who would choose to live longer if they could not do so independently. With this in mind, the program presented here is designed to increase your functional capacity, not just help you live longer. After all, life should be *lived* with vitality and filled with purpose, not merely endured.

As you go about improving your level of fitness, you will discover a great deal about yourself in the process. In order to improve how you look and feel, you must be willing to change your lifestyle. While lifestyle changes can be hard the rewards will far outweigh the cost.

To change anything in life, be it your financial status, your relationships, or your body, you must first change your mind. That is why this program focuses first on mental conditioning, *before* tackling physical conditioning.

This program will teach you:

- ➢ The power of goal setting and visualization and how to apply them to your fitness goals

- ➢ Four key components to activity and how they are interrelated

- ➢ Real-Life exercises that will fit into the busiest schedules

- ➢ Ten Keys to Fueling Your Body Right

- ➢ How to put the plan in action and you on a path toward optimal health

Now, let's get started by looking at one of the most powerful tools you will ever use in your life.

CHAPTER 1

SMART GOALS

The Power of Goal Setting

It is believed that less than ten percent of the American population has written goals. Yet those who do, business people like Bill Gates, motivational speakers such as Mark Victor Hansen and athletes like Russell Wilson achieve far more than those of us that do not have written goals.

Consider that, as a teenager Bill Gates had a vision that every business and household should have a computer. Together with Paul Allen he started *Microsoft* in 1975 and by the mid-eighties began to see his vision for a simple operating system come into focus with the launch of *Windows*.

Today, his ultimate goal is becoming a reality, as computers are more prevalent in homes and businesses than ever before. Increasingly within the United States most homes have at least one computer, and when it comes to business, few today would even consider operating without one. If not for his **vision,** it's unlikely personal computers would be as commonplace as they are today, and he surely would not be the richest man in the world.

Regardless of what you would like to achieve in your lifetime the simple fact is: to accomplish anything of significance in life requires careful planning, focused actions and constant effort directed toward the achievement of a goal. Achieving and maintaining a healthy body is no different.

When you consider that, without your health nothing else matters, there are few conditions of greater importance than fitness. You probably have some idea about the level of fitness you want to achieve, although right now your images of fitness are just dreams. In order to make your dreams reality you must set clear, specific goals.

Goal setting is one of the most powerful tools you will ever use in your life!

My first truly memorable experience with goal setting was through sports. My football coach decided that a lack of goals was the missing link in our quest for the championship, and he was determined to change that. Preceding my senior year in high school, our coaches attended a seminar conducted by Lou Tice of *The Pacific Institute*. The program, called *Thought Patterns for Winners,* taught us how to use goal setting and visualization as tools to condition our minds.

We started the program during the summer with a weekend retreat. We came together as a team and learned the mechanics of goal setting and why it works (more on this subject later). Each day we would meet as a team, discuss what we wanted to accomplish and then set goals for the season. Our ultimate goal was to win the conference championship.

Following the team's goal setting sessions, my teammates and I practiced and worked out at a higher level than we ever had before. We were now driven by a common purpose and a renewed sense of enthusiasm. There was a completely different attitude when compared to the year before, and I knew that we would compete at a much higher level.

We started the season by crushing our first opponent 28 – 0. Although we continued to play well throughout most of the season, we didn't win the championship. We lost to the eventual conference champions by 3 points, a team that we had not expected to be competitive.

I recall reviewing my *Thought Patterns for Winners* notebook after the season, and found that we defeated every team we focused on. The problem was, the best team in our conference that year was one of the worst the year before. In fact, the conference champions were one of only two teams we had defeated the previous season. Every team that we defeated mentally, in our mind's eye, we later defeated on the field of play. But those teams we left out, the ones we expected to beat, defeated us. Two of the games we lost by 3 points and the other by 7. Had we practiced goal setting and visualization in preparation for these games there is no doubt in my mind we would have gone undefeated.

Why Not You?

If goal setting is so wonderful, why is it not more common? What is keeping us from setting goals so that we can achieve more? There are a number of reasons people do not set goals.

Three main reasons people do not set goals are:

1. We lack a clear understanding as to why goals are important.
2. We do not know how to go about it.
3. We fear the unknown and the possibility of failure.

Here is a closer look at why most of us do not set goals:

- We lack a clear understanding as to why goals are important. During our younger years' life was planned out for us, the classes we needed to take, our schedules, even the deadlines for getting assignments done were all set. Later, as adults we become captains of our own ship and suddenly it is up to us to decide which way to go in life. Unfortunately, it is at this point that we find out how ill prepared we are to manage our own lives and the one thing that can help us, goal setting…

- We do not know how to go about it: Although some of us are exposed to goal setting in school, it is rarely taught to any great extent or with any real follow-up. Without a clear understanding of how to set and achieve a goal it is unlikely to be practiced. Even if you were exposed to goal setting in greater detail, you may avoid the process altogether due to a common condition known as...

- A fear of failure: Most of us prefer to stay in our comfort zone rather than risk failure. In an uncertain world we look for something to cling to, something familiar. This is a big mistake because change is inevitable. We cannot stand still in life, either we are moving forward or we are getting passed by. The reality is that without taking calculated risks we can be assured a life of mediocrity.

When you take a look at history you will find those who achieved excellence experienced various setbacks along the way. In fact, the challenges they faced served as valuable lessons and sources of motivation for their future success.

Here are a few examples:
- o Imagine one of the greatest basketball players of all time being cut from his high school basketball team. Here is the story told by Bob Greene in *Reader's Digest*: One November night, **Michael Jordan** and I found ourselves alone, and he told me about being cut as a sophomore from his high-school basketball team in Wilmington, N.C. "The day the cut list was going up, a friend—Leroy Smith—and I went to the gym to look together," Jordan recalled. "If your name was on the list, you made the team. Leroy's name was there, and mine wasn't. I went through the day numb. After school, I hurried home, closed the door to my room and cried so hard. It was all I wanted—to play on that team."

Rather than getting down on himself and giving up, he used this experience as motivation to spur him on. Jordan went on to say, "Whenever I was working out and got tired and figured I ought to stop, I'd close my eyes and see that list in the locker room without my name on it and that usually got me going again."

o   According to Charles Reichblum's, *Knowledge in a Nutshell*, one of the greatest scientists of all time, **Albert Einstein,** did poorly in elementary school and even failed his first college entrance exam at Zurich Polytechnic.

It is important to note, however, he did not do poorly in all subjects, and in fact excelled in mathematics. Apparently, he hated the elementary school he attended because his classes were based on memorization and obedience. He was more interested in learning *why* things were so. It was not until he focused his energies proving various theories through mathematics and physics that he began to excel.

o   **Henry Ford** is quoted as saying "Failure is only the opportunity to begin again more intelligently." He knew this to be true because the automobile manufacturer's first two companies failed. His first company filed for bankruptcy and the second ended because of a disagreement with his business partner. In June 1903, at the age of 40, he created a third company, the Ford Motor Company with a cash investment of $28,000.00.

By July of 1903 the bank balance had dwindled to $223.65, but then Ford sold its first car, and as they say, the rest is history.

As these three famous people have shown, you only fail if you stop trying.

Bridging the Gap

You may be familiar with the saying: "knowledge is power." The truth, as Napoleon Hill points out in his bestselling book, *Think and Grow Rich,* is that, "Knowledge is only *potential* power." You can have all the knowledge in the world, however until you apply that knowledge it is useless. The difference between succeeding or failing in life today, is less a question of knowing what to do, than it is doing what you already know.

Consider what you already know about how to increase your level of physical activity. Things like walking more and driving less, climbing the stairs instead of using the elevator, or even working in your yard. Now compare what you know you *should* do to what you actually do each day. What makes it so difficult to *just do it*? Is it a lack of information? Probably not, in fact information overload is a more likely contributor to your dilemma. Between your computer, smart phone, television, magazines, and the radio the sheer volume of information we are inundated with each day boggles the mind. In our fast-paced lives, the difficulty lies in the ability to stay focused on the most important task at any given moment, and then to make performing that task as routine as brushing your teeth. Goal setting will get you focused on the direction you wish to go and bridge the gap between the *knowing* and the *doing* in your life.

Why Goal Setting Works

Before we go into the "how-to" of goal setting, it is important for you to understand the science behind why goal setting works. That way you can apply these principles with confidence, knowing that your goal setting efforts will be fruitful.

A great deal of research has been done with regard to how our mind works. Many of the conclusions may be found in Dr. Maxwell Maltz's timeless classic *Psycho-Cybernetics*, first published back in 1960. His work demonstrated one undeniable fact: we become what we think about. In other words, you are who you are today because of the thoughts that dominate your mind. Even King Solomon, considered the wisest man in the land said:

"Keep your heart with all diligence, for out of it spring the issues of life." Proverbs 4:23 NKJV

Your mind is divided into two main parts: *conscious* and *subconscious*. Your conscious mind distinguishes between what is real and what is imaginary. Reason and logic are the stuff of our conscious mind. On the other hand, your subconscious mind cannot tell the difference between a real or imaginary experience. In addition, your subconscious never takes even a moment off, recording information continually, 24 hours a day, 365 days a year. Everything you see, hear, taste, touch, smell, and even dream about gets imprinted on your mind.

There seems to be little research on exactly how many thoughts you have each day. Since much of our thinking happens at a subconscious level it makes it particularly difficult to count a person's thoughts. One of the few sources I found, *The National Science Foundation*, has determined the average person has about 12,000 thoughts per day while awake, with deep

deep thinkers having up to 50,000 thoughts every day. That equates to between 360,000 - 1.5 million thoughts per month, 4.5 - 20 million every year.

Sadly, for many of us, the majority of these thoughts are negative. One reason for this is that we are bombarded with negative messages through the media every day. Just log into your favorite news site and read the headlines or switch on the news and take note of the lead story – bad news no doubt.

Here are some examples of recent headlines:
- **Only 12 years to limit climate change before catastrophe**
- **Too much screen time has lasting consequences**
- **What I Wish I Had Known About Marriage**

Advertising agencies and media moguls are well aware of one important fact, that when given the choice with regards to enjoying pleasurable thoughts versus the removal of pain, the brain is wired to remove pain first. This is a **survival instinct**, forcing us to deal with any potentially dangerous situations first, before thinking about anything else.

Negative information gets our attention. We want to know what's happening so we can avoid any potential problems. Even the weather report works this way. If the weather is particularly extreme—be it too hot, too cold, too windy or wet—we want to know about it so we can avoid it. If a storm blows in, it's a lead story; if it's a sunny day with mild temperatures, the weather report is done at the end of the broadcast.

Besides messages from the media, the people with whom we associate also impact us. Since the majority of messages the average person takes in each day are negative, it is likely they will in turn spew out negativity. This is an important reason why you should carefully choose the people with whom you associate.

Amazingly, of the 12,000 – 50,000 thoughts you have each day, **95 – 98% of them are the same ones you had yesterday**. When you consider this high percentage, it is no wonder that we truly are creatures of habit.

These numbers illustrate the importance of paying attention to the things that we input into our super-computer like minds. When it comes to our thought patterns the **GIGO** principle applies: **G**ood **I**n, **G**ood **O**ut or **G**arbage **I**n, **G**arbage **O**ut. Thankfully we all have a choice as to what to fill our minds with. We decide what to read, watch on television, listen to on the radio, and whose company to keep. We either funnel positive messages into our minds leading towards the achievement of our goals, or by default the negative messages we are exposed to lead us away from our desired path.

The Process of Goal Setting

Now that you know why goal setting is important and how it works, let's take a closer look at the process of setting a goal. Keep in mind, goal setting is a skill, and like any other skill it takes time to learn. Be patient, yet persistent in your goal setting efforts, as the positive effects will be well worth it.

One very important part of the goal setting process goals is that **they must be written down**. If your goals are not in writing, they are just dreams. Dreams are great for creating ideas and deciding what you want to achieve in life; however, dreams don't just *come true* by chance. You have to take *action* to turn fantasy into reality.

Writing down your goals accomplishes the following important steps:

1. **Create a Plan** – As the saying goes "If you fail to plan, you plan to fail." A plan will give you a distinct direction in which to work toward your goals, making you more efficient and keeping you on track.

2. **Make a Commitment** – It is one thing to think or say you are going to do something. When you put it in writing, it becomes a personal contract.

3. **Establish a Record** – Writing down your goals allows you learn from past experiences, revisit your success, and will in turn breed further achievements.

When you write down your goals make sure they are:

➤ Positive!! Since we become what we think about, it is important to focus on what you want, not what you don't want in life.

> Example: Write: "I am lean." Don't write: "I am not fat."

> Since our subconscious mind cannot tell the difference between an imaginary and **actual experience** when it comes to your goals:

> **"If it's believable, then it's achievable."**

➤ SMART – There are different variations to the SMART goal setting acronym. The combination that I have found most useful is:

Specific, **M**easurable, **A**ction-Oriented, **R**ealistic and **T**angible

Here is an overview of the component parts of SMART. You will find many of the components overlap. Each part is important, both individually and as a whole.

<u>S</u>pecific

The more specific your goals are, the better chance you have of reaching them. Think in terms of the five **W**'s as you answer these important questions.

- **Who** is involved?
- **What** do I want to accomplish?
- **When** as in timeframe (long-term, intermediate, short-term).
- **Where** do I want to see my results?
- **Why** it is important to me? (The "Why" is very important because when you are passionate about your goals you are more likely to achieve them).

<u>M</u>easurable

By setting measurable goals (how much? or how many?) you are able to monitor your progress. Monitoring your progress is key so that you can adjust your actions according to the results you are achieving.

<u>A</u>ction – Oriented

What things need to be done to reach your goals? Excellence does not just happen; **you** have to **make it** happen. Set your goals in line with your level of passion to reach them and then take *action* on the things that need to get done each day.

Realistic

There is no such thing as an unrealistic goal, just unrealistic time frames. Consider where you are now and where you want to be, then set goals for gradual, yet steady progress.

Tangible

Setting tangible goals makes it easier to **visualize** your success. If you can taste, touch, smell, see, or hear your goal it is tangible.

When setting your goals, it is important to compare to your own best self, not others. If you compare yourself to others, you will **never** be satisfied. When a client tells me, they want to look or be like someone else, I simply say, "You do not have their parents." While there is nothing wrong with having role models, remember that genetics always play a role. Do not get too caught up in the comparison game, but rather consider where **you** are now... and where **you** want to go.

Set goals in every area of your life, both personally and professionally. Although we will be discussing goal setting with regard to fitness, these principles should be applied to all aspects of your life. After all, mental, physical, and spiritual fitness, together with a productive career and healthy family life are all interconnected. Without one, the others are of little importance. Look to strike a balance in your life by considering what is most important to you and then set your goals accordingly.

Before we set some fitness goals, let's first consider four key components of an activity program.

CHAPTER 2
FITT
PRINCIPLES

FITT COMPONENTS

When beginning an activity program, there are a few things you must decide: namely how often, how hard, how long, and what type of activity you should do? These are the components of the acronym **FITT** (**F**requency, **I**ntensity, **T**ime, and **T**ype).

While we will be looking at each component separately, we must also consider how one factor affects the other. For example, the **intensity** level of an activity will have a direct effect on the length of **time** you can continue and the **frequency** that specific activity should be performed.

For example, when my athletes perform 40-yard wind sprints they are generally given two minutes or more to recover between sets. If they are running a longer distance, say 400 meters, their rest period between sets will often last 90 seconds or less. Following wind sprints or hard interval training sessions, the participants will often need more recover days before repeating an intense training session.

Frequency

The human body is designed to be *active*. Primitive man and woman did not wake-up each day and ponder *if* they would hunt and gather food, build their shelter or protect their territory. These were essential actions that required their energy **every day**. In addition, the men had to take care of the time-honored tradition their wives had likely prepared for them:

> HONEY- DO LIST
>
> 1. Fix the leaky roof.
> 2. Re-tie the loose rope swing.
> 3. Teach junior how to hunt and fish.

While in today's modern society you do not have to be active to survive, you do need to be active to achieve **optimal health** and truly *live* life. The idea is to schedule activity into your life on a **daily** basis. Physical activity needs to become as common as your other daily actions, like brushing your teeth and taking a shower for example. Think about it. At what point in life do we say, "I've done enough tooth brushing, I am done with this." The answer of course is never. The same can be said for exercise.

Newton's first law, *the law of motion* applies here. You will find that the more active you are, the easier it is to remain in that condition, while the less you do the greater effort required to get started. Our body's condition comes down to one basic law, the law of use: "**Use it or lose it.**"

<u>I</u>ntensity

When discussing **how hard** to exercise, one of the first things I tell my clients is "you have the rest of your life to get fit." If you have become deconditioned, keep in mind that has occurred over time: weeks, months, possibly even years to reach your present condition. If you are like most people, you want results **fast**. There are many programs that take advantage of this fact and promote their programs with slick advertising campaigns, "Lose 30 pounds in 30 days," "Reshape your thighs in 7 days" or "Build massive shoulders in just two weeks."

With regard to weight loss, you may be able to in fact lose 30 pounds in 30 days, but the question is, at what cost? These programs should be avoided for two main reasons:

1. They are too restrictive to follow for life and therefore do not provide lasting results.
2. Crash diets produce rapid weight loss, much of which is muscle. This slows your metabolism and causes you to regain the weight.

The fact is, good things take time, including improving your fitness level. Few people realize that your fitness level does not actually improve while you are exercising. This is the stress or resistance phase. Your fitness level actually improves during the recovery period, as your body adapts. Therefore, the right amount of activity, intermixed with the right amount of rest, will produce the best results.

With this in mind, forget the adage "No pain, No gain." Although some muscle soreness is expected, there is no reason why you should be in extreme pain in the days following your sessions. Trust me, I've been there. It is easy, particularly in a competitive environment, to overdo it. I can remember a few different occasions where sitting down and walking, particularly up and down stairs, was very painful. Just keep in mind; gradual steady progress is the best approach for a lifetime of health and fitness.

If you find yourself very sore the day or days following your workout, do not stop exercising, as this will delay your progress. Just decrease the intensity level of your sessions until the soreness subsides. Spend 5 to 10 minutes doing a variety of the movements presented in the program followed by some light stretching.

Since you will be active daily, your intensity level cannot always be at its maximum. The best strategy includes a mixture of hard, moderate and easy (active recovery) days throughout the week. Typically, I have my athletes mix in some active recovery every third or fourth day.

Everyone is different when it comes to how his or her body responds to exercise. There are a number of factors that affect recovery: age, diet, the amount of sleep you get each night to name a few. As we age our bodies recover slower. You will find out what works best for you over time and adjust your lifestyle accordingly.

We will look at intensity in greater detail later, for now let's check the...

<u>T</u>ime

When deciding how much time to be active each day, there are a few things to consider. Although your goals and schedule will dictate the amount of time in the end, a minimum of 30 minutes per day is recommended for general fitness. Most likely you will find yourself dedicating more time to your activity as your fitness improves. When it comes to activity, most authorities, such as **The American College of Sports Medicine,** agree, **"*Some* is better than *none,* and *more* is better than *some*."**

Your activity does not have to be done continuously as once thought. Mix in some activity throughout the day, approximately 10 to 15 minutes each session, morning, afternoon and evening. Build up to at least one session of 45 to 60 minutes per week. Weekends are often a good time for this as you may have fewer commitments on these days.

Longer workouts allow you to develop greater endurance, incorporate a variety of movements and spend more time cooling down and stretching out. The only reason you would need to exercise longer than 60 minutes would be to burn additional calories or if you were training for a specific event such as a long hike or marathon.

Now that we have decided how often, how hard, and how long you should be active, let's now consider what kind of activity I recommend and why.

<u>T</u>ype

It is difficult to say that one activity is better than another one, let alone to say one is "The Best." While every form of exercise has value, no matter how beneficial it may be, without regular practice it is of little worth. Remember, the number one reason people give for not being more active is "I don't have time" therefore, the time factor must be considered.

In order to be considered the best, from my perspective it should meet the following criteria:

- Appropriate for all ages and fitness levels.

- Can be done anywhere: in your home, at the park, on the beach, or even at the local fitness or recreation center.

- Requires little or no equipment.

- Easy to learn proper technique.

- Time efficient, total body workout in as little as 10 minutes.

- Enough variation to keep you from getting bored.

- Challenging enough to keep you motivated for a lifetime.

- Targets the main components of total body fitness: body composition, muscular strength, muscular endurance, balance and flexibility.

- Can do it alone, with a buddy or even in a group.

- Weather proof.

- Complements all other forms of activity.

The only activity that I have found to meet all of these requirements is... bodyweight exercises. Does that mean that all other forms of activity are useless? No, in fact you will find a variety of other activities recommended in this program. So, if you like to run, cycle, hike, play racket sports, or any other form of physical activity, by all means continue doing it. Just do it in conjunction with the exercises taught in this program. Besides, unless you are an exception, it is unlikely you are doing these activities on a daily basis.

Now that you have a basic understanding of both SMART GOALS and FITT PRINCIPLES let's get into greater detail of the program, first with regard to goal setting and then the conditioning program.

CHAPTER 3
SETTING YOUR FITNESS GOALS

The Key to Your Success

How many times have you started an exercise program vowing that "this time I am really going to stick with it?" Maybe this is your first quest for fitness, or perhaps you are *beginning* again. Either way, if you are like most people, you will jump right into your program without giving much thought to what it is you want to achieve. And if there is some thought given, it is often too vague to have any real impact. If you ask the average person *why* they have started to exercise, they'll likely say, "I want to lose *some* weight." Or you might hear, "I have to *get in shape*." Neither of these reasons could pass as a goal and therefore are unlikely to motivate them beyond a few days or possibly a week.

Whatever reasons you may have for improving your fitness level, the key to your success resides between your ears. This is true because, as we learned in CHAPTER 1, SMART GOALS, when you condition your mind, your body will follow.

Remember these two undeniable facts:

1. Your subconscious mind (internal computer) does not know the difference between an actual and imagined experience.

2. You become what you think about.

When you set your goals, make sure to set big ones as, **big goals motivate**. If your goals are not big enough, there may not be enough reasons **why** to keep you going. As a leading self-improvement expert, Jim Rohn says, "When the **why** gets bigger, the **how** gets easier."

Setting big goals can be intimidating. To overcome your fear, think of the age-old adage, "How do you eat an elephant?" The answer is, "one bite at a time." When you think of the entire task your goal represents, possibly losing 60 pounds or running a marathon, it looks huge. When you break it up into smaller, "bite sized" pieces, like losing 2 pounds per week or increasing your mileage totals by 10 – 15% per week it becomes more manageable.

Focusing on the weight loss goal, losing 60 pounds of body fat, break it down into weekly and monthly targets. With a weekly goal of 2 pounds as you get started, then aim for averaging between 1 – 2 pounds of fat loss per week or about 6 pounds a month. Continuing on this path, losing 6 pounds each month, you will have lost 60 pounds in ten months.

To make all of your goals more manageable, break them down into various time frames as these:

- Short-term goal (1-month)
- Intermediate goal (3 – 6 months)
- Long-term goal (1-year)
- Ultimate Long-term goal (3 – 5 years)

Life is a journey and no matter what the length of the trip is, it begins with one step. Keep your big goals in front of you for inspiration but focus your efforts on what you can do each day to bring you closer to your dreams.

Since many people today are fighting *the battle of the bulge,* I have selected a fat loss goal to serve as an example.

Sample Goal – Fat Loss

Goal setting is a proven method for making the seemingly impossible, possible. Be sure to write your goals with faith that they will be achieved. One way to express this faith is to state your goals with **positive emotion** for the things you are going to do, be or have, in this case a leaner body.

Reaching 12% bodyfat **feels great**...

and then continue with the **SMART** components:

Specific

> **Who**, **what**, **when**, **where** and **why**
>
> **Reaching 12% body fat on August 18, 2020 feels great! My new body shape allows me to fit into clothes I have not been able to wear in years**.

Measurable

> Reaching **12% body fat**... Your **body fat percentage** is a common and **objective** way to express your body composition. In order for something to be measurable it must be based on objective facts and figures, not subjective thoughts and feelings.

Action-Oriented You will learn more about the activity and nutritional plans mentioned here in greater detail in ensuing chapters. The following serve only as examples for now.

Action Plan – Activity

- I am active in the morning, afternoon and an evening for at least 10 minutes each session or a minimum of 30 minutes of continuous activity most days of the week (4 – 6 days/week).
- Throughout each day I stay active by walking, climbing the stairs and doing things around school, work or home together with any other activity that keeps me moving.
- At least once a week, I am active working in the yard or recreating in my favorite sport.

Action Plan – Nutritional

- I am thankful for the abundance of natural foods I am eating each day. My body is well nourished, and I feel energized.
- I eat in a way that controls my blood sugar level, keeping my sugar and starchy carbohydrate intake to a minimum.

Realistic

Reaching **12% body fat on August 18th, 2020**... The amount of fat loss you wish to achieve represents only part of insuring your goal is realistic. The date by which you plan to reach your goal is an equally important factor. While obtaining a particular percentage of body fat may be realistic, is the amount of time you have allotted sufficient to do so healthfully? A reasonable rate of fat loss is between 0.5 – 0.7% of your body fat or about 1 – 2 pounds (0.5 – 0.8 kilos) of fat per week. Although you may lose a bit more some weeks, aim for steady, consistent fat loss within this range until you reach your goal.

Tangible

Remember, the tangible part of your goal has to do with your senses. With a fat loss goal, you can definitely **see** and **feel** the difference your new shape will make.

Reaching 12% body fat on August 18, 2020 feels great! My new body shape allows me to **fit into cloths** I have not been able to wear in years.

The tangible aspects of your goals become particularly useful as you apply the power of…

Visualization

Earlier I stated, "Goal setting is one of the most powerful tools you will ever use in your life." And while this is true, without the use of visualization your goals will be less likely to be achieved. If you cannot see your desired self in your mind's eye (imagination), then the habits necessary to move from your current to your desired condition will be inhibited.

Remember, one of the keys when writing down your goals is to state what you want to achieve, not what you don't want. Think of your dreams, how real do they seem before you wake up? Without a conscious awareness they seem as real as any other experience you've had. It is only after you wake up in a sweat that you realize "oh no" or "whew," it was only a dream.

Since it is within a dream state that your visualization exercises will be most effective, the best time to practice is in the morning as you are in an alpha state, a dream like condition that makes your mind more receptive to new ideas. Spend some time each day, at least 5 minutes in the morning and at night visualizing the achievement of your goals.

To make your mental practice more effective at any other time of the day enter an alpha state through a relaxation exercise like this:

- Find a warm, quiet place where you can relax and focus your mind.

- Sit down in a comfortable position.

- Now focus on your breath: inhale deeply through your nose feeling your belly rise, hold it for two seconds then exhale slowly through your mouth saying *ah*. Continue this breathing exercise until you are completely relaxed.

Once you have quieted your mind, try this visualization exercise:

- See yourself waking up early, excited to begin a new day.

- Smell the aroma and taste the flavor of your favorite pre-activity snack and feel the energy it provides.

- Feel your body warm-up as you begin your movements.

- Notice how good you feel after completing your morning activity session.

- Continue to picture yourself living healthfully throughout the day, eating well and keeping your body moving.

- Feel the difference your new, fit body has made in your life.

When you practice visualization exercises regularly, it will have a profound effect on your mind-set, and therefore your future actions. You will find yourself moving away from undesirable behavior and moving toward the actions necessary to achieve your goals.

A *New* You

Through this process of goal setting and visualization you are creating a new "self-image." Your self-image is developed over time, from the people that impacted your life to the experiences you've had. Your self-image may be a limiting belief such as, "I will never be lean" or "I will always be broke." But your self-image can also become, "I am lean and fit" or "I am financially successful." You can create the life that you want through your thoughts and actions that are in alignment with your goals. As a wise person once said, "Act as though I am and I will be."

Setting Your Goals

For your goals to have maximum effect it is important that they are in alignment with your other life purposes and are rooted in good intentions. As you work towards a worthy goal, sometimes you'll experience various setbacks. If you've set a fitness-based goal you may experience an injury or catch a cold. Challenges are inevitable. Continue to work through these temporary setbacks, and remember, ultimately God is in control.

> **"Many are the plans in the mind of a man, but it is the purpose of the Lord that will stand." Proverbs 19:21 ESV**

Below I have provided a few sample goals, it is up to you to decide what you want to achieve and more importantly to what lengths you are willing to go to get there. When it comes to setting fitness goals, the possibilities are virtually limitless.

To narrow your focus, start with these three categories:

1. Number of repetitions completed for your favorite exercise.
2. Time/Distance goal for one of the *A to B with a Purpose* activities.
3. Complete a specific event such as a 5-kilometer fun run, triathlon, or even climb a mountain.

Here is another sample goal using one of the three examples above:

Beginning with **positive emotion**…

I am **joyful…**and then continue with the **SMART** components:

Specific

> **Who, what, when, where** and **why**?
>
> **I am** joyful to **reach the summit of Mount Olympus on September 15, 2020, improving my endurance, balance and coordination**.

Measurable

> To reach **the summit of Mount Olympus** (measurable distance).

Action-Oriented (The following action plans serves only as an example).

> Action Plan – Activity
>
> - My activity sessions are 30 – 60 minutes of continuous movement most days of the week with a least one longer session increasing in length from 60 minutes building to 120 minutes.
> - At least once a week, I am hiking on increasingly difficult terrain and longer distances.

Action Plan – Nutritional

- I eat healthfully each day, meeting my energy requirements and maintaining a strong, healthy body.
- I eat various dry, portable foods during my training to find out what foods I find easier to digest while climbing.

Realistic

I am joyful to **reach the summit of Mount Olympus on September 15, 2020.** The difficulty of the climb and the date which you plan to reach the summit factor into whether it is a realistic goal. While climbing Mount Olympus may be a realistic goal, do you have adequate time to prepare for it by September 15, 2020?

Tangible

I am joyful to reach the summit of Mount Olympus on September 15, 2020, **improving my endurance, balance and coordination**.

Before moving on, take some time and practice writing 1 – 3 of your fitness goals in the space provided in appendix A. Once you have set a few goals, begin to practice visualization, and then tonight before you go to sleep practice it again. The more you practice, the greater chance you have of turning your dreams into reality.

CHAPTER 4
REAL-LIFE
CONDITIONING

<u>**Let's Get Physical**</u>

Now that you have your mental conditioning program started, it is time to *get physical*. Before you get started on the program here are some of the particulars.

You are not likely to find this Real-Life Conditioning Program handed out at your local gym, and you won't find it in the glossy fitness magazines either. This program will prepare you to meet the physical demands, not just of everyday life, but will allow you to truly live your life to the fullest.

I could tell you to just follow the program because it works, as that's true. But that might not be enough for some of you. If you're like me, you want to know why. When you know *why* something works, you can then dive in with confidence knowing that your time will be well spent.

Here are three important reasons why this program works:

1. Real-Life Movements – Consider how we move each day: sitting, standing, walking, squatting, pushing and pulling. All of these actions require the use of your muscles through multiple joints moving our body as a unit. Yet a large percentage of the exercising public is taught to focus on one muscle or muscle group at a time, often working different body parts on different days.

   Although there is no single *right* way to exercise, since our body functions as a unit during day-to-day activities, it makes sense that we practice in this way.

2. Utilizes a Variety of Energy Systems – There are times when we have to work very hard for brief periods of time. There are also occasions where we have to work at a more moderate intensity for longer

periods. This program taps into both energy systems and allows your body to adapt in a way that aligns with your lifestyle.

3. Gradual, Steady Progress – The human body is an amazing machine that gets more efficient with use. When you apply the principles taught in this program your fitness will improve gradually. As you improve you can alter the FITT components to achieve your desired fitness level.

Recording Your Sessions

It is important that you record your activity sessions accurately. By doing this you are accomplishing a few things. First of all, you are documenting what you have done. This is a positive thing, in and of itself, as keeping a journal will reaffirm what you have accomplished. In addition, it allows you to compare past sessions with your current level, clearly showing your progress. Finally, it helps you plan future sessions based on past performances and your current condition, be it well rested or fatigued.

Sample recording forms are provided in the appendix. These will help you keep track of each session's results: exercises performed, amount of weight lifted, number of repetitions completed, and the amount of time within an activity. You will also find a place to record your total time exercised and average heart rate (heart rate monitor required) during your *A to B with a Purpose* sessions.

How About Stretching?

Many people ask if they should stretch **before** they exercise, largely because that's what we were taught as kids and even today by some fitness *experts*. And while I highly recommend stretching, I find the passive, easy type of stretching most of us are familiar more beneficial at the end of your activity session, as part of a cool-down.

Every type of exercise incorporates some form of stretching, typically in a dynamic fashion as we flex and extend our muscles throughout the movement. Remember: one of the many benefits of Body Weight Exercises is that they simultaneously develop, balance, strength, endurance and flexibility.

The program presented here contains controlled movements that do not require a great deal of stretching before you begin. If you are exercising first thing in the morning you may find yourself a bit tight. If this is the case, you will need to do an active warm-up. I have included a few movements to get you going in the program section below.

A Word About Exercise Equipment

A few of the exercises contained within this program require various apparatus, weights and resistance bands for example. I have made the foundation of this program body weight exercises for reasons given earlier within chapter 2. Thankfully, this eliminates the need for a great deal of equipment that is required with most other programs. It does not, however, eliminate the need for a few key items.

Weight is needed for the various lifting exercises and depending on where you plan to do your program you may need to purchase some form of cardiovascular equipment (treadmill, cycle, rower, etc.). If you are resourceful, you may be able to utilize a few things around the house. You can fill up plastic 1-gallon milk cartons with sand or grab some canned food for weight. You also may have a flight of stairs or sturdy bench in your home that you can use for climbing or stepping activity.

Words of caution as you look for ways to improvise. Do not use anything that is suspect with regard to its condition. A wobbly bench, for example could cause you to fall. It is not worth saving a few bucks and risking injury in the process. After all, this program is supposed to help you avoid the hospital, not send you there.

Depending on the climate and air quality where you live, you may want to invest in some indoor exercise equipment. Like most things, when it comes to exercise equipment, you really do get what you pay for. Don't let slick sales representatives or fancy advertising fool you. Cheap exercise equipment is no bargain. It will not hold up well to regular use, and the quality of the experience will be compromised by annoyances like wobbly seats, squeaks, or slipping treadmill belts.

The Movements

The Real-Life Conditioning exercises in this program are a starting point from which to work and by no means represent an exhaustive list. The variety of exercises available and the combinations that they may be used is limited only by one's imagination.

The exercises presented here are of great value, if done properly. However, if you just go through the motions, without attention to how your body feels throughout the movement, you will miss out on many of their benefits. For this reason, become familiar with each exercise first before proceeding onward. Think quality, not quantity at the beginning, and then work on increasing volume and intensity.

Types of Muscular Contractions

Our muscles contract in three distinct ways as we go about our daily lives. By gaining a greater understanding of each type of contraction, you can then alter your range of motion and speed of each movement as needed.

Isometric – An *Isometric* contraction is when the muscles contract, but there is no change in the angle of the joint. Your muscles contract in an isometric manner to maintain your posture and stabilize your body during various positions and movements. Isometric contractions are very effective at increasing muscular strength and will be used when performing a larger number of dynamic movements proves difficult.

Eccentric – An *Eccentric* contraction is when the muscles contract as two points move further apart. Eccentric contractions help to control your body in motion, particularly during deceleration, such as walking down a flight of stairs or walking/running downhill.

As you perform the exercises presented here make a point of using your muscles to lower the weight under control, generally on a 3 – 4 second count. This will accentuate the eccentric contraction so that you will get the most from each exercise. As a variation, lengthen the amount of time in the lowering phase to further emphasize the eccentric contraction.

Concentric – A *Concentric* contraction is when the muscles contract to bring two points closer together. Concentric contractions occur as we lift something, such as our body weight or an external object (weight).
Avoid fast, jerky actions as you perform the lifting phase of the exercises. Move smoothly and under control raising the weight on about a 2 to 4 second count. You may also lengthen the amount of time in the "lifting" phase of the movement, reducing momentum and increasing the difficulty of the exercise.

Here are examples of each type of muscular contraction:

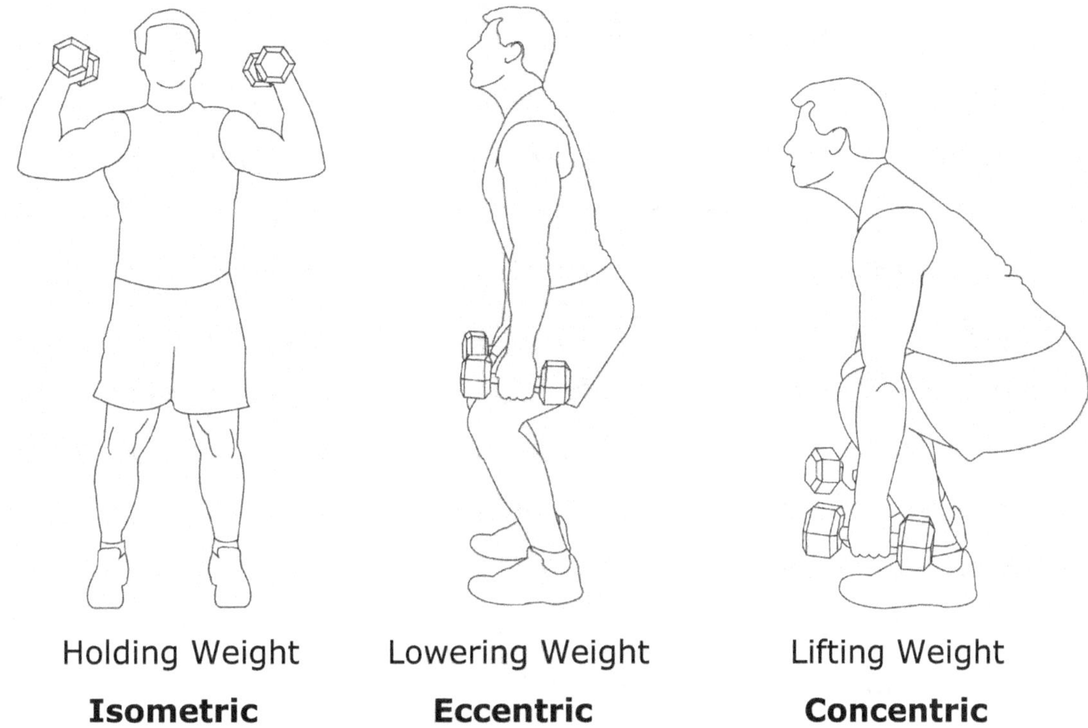

Holding Weight

Isometric

Lowering Weight

Eccentric

Lifting Weight

Concentric

<u>Breathing</u>

Although our bodies breathe automatically, the quality of our breathing patterns is not always the best. Day-to-day stresses, poor posture and our general lack of fitness contribute to a restricted flow of air in and out of our lungs.

Taking in oxygen and expelling carbon dioxide (breathing) is a fundamental part of life and is therefore emphasized in this program. In fact, your breathing should be a focal point rather than an afterthought during these movements. By focusing on your breathing, you will be able to maximize your efforts and get the most out of your sessions.

<u>**Strength/Endurance**</u>

Two extreme examples of *fitness*, a Power Lifter and a Marathoner speak volumes with regard to energy demands. The former is capable of performing at a high intensity for short periods of time, while the latter can go for hours while maintaining a relatively low intensity level. It is physiologically impossible to be successful at both power lifting *and* long distance running at the same time. And although neither of these extremes may be something you wish to emulate; you can likely appreciate the differences with regard to the energy each athlete requires.

Most activities in everyday life require a combination of both strength and endurance. Be it a box full of books or your expanding backpack, there are times when you need to pick up and carry something heavy. And when it comes to stamina, every day is a marathon of sorts. You're up early and on the go all day, rushing from one meeting or class to the next, tackling your "to do's." Endurance is *definitely* a factor.

This program will give you the strength and endurance necessary to handle daily physical challenges with enough energy left over for leisure time pursuits or to meet any emergency demands.

In order to achieve overall fitness this program combines:

- The resistance training exercises mentioned above.

- Moderate to high intensity cardiovascular "aerobic" activity, referred to as A to B with a purpose.

A to B with a Purpose

In addition to the various squatting, lifting, pushing and pulling movements, our bodies are also designed to move us from one place to another, without the use of a motor! With this in mind, to achieve optimal health we should incorporate at least one, or preferably a combination of these movements into our daily routine: brisk walking, running, cycling, rowing and swimming.

Walking

Walking is an excellent form of exercise, for a variety of reasons. One reason is its weight bearing nature. Weight bearing exercise is important to help us build and maintain bone mass, fighting off osteoporosis (brittle bone disease). Walking can be done almost anywhere, as all that it requires is comfortable shoes, proper clothing for the climate and a safe environment.

In order for walking to be an effective form of exercise, it must be done briskly, particularly if you are on a flat surface. Good form involves standing up tall, stepping quickly and pumping your arms to help move you forward at a faster pace. Aim for 3.5 – 4.0 mph or 5.0 – 6.5 km/hour.

Walking uphill or hiking is even better as this increases the amount of energy you will expend. Start with some easy climbs and gradually add onto the length and difficultly of the slope. When coming back downhill, be sure-footed and control your speed to help maintain your balance.

Running

Running is an exceptional form of exercise for many of the same reasons as walking, specifically its weight bearing nature and convenience. In addition, the flight phase of running creates a feeling which many people find euphoric, known as a *runner's high*.

Running is not for everyone though, as the impact can be too jarring for many people. If you have orthopedic issues in your low back, hips, knees or ankles, running may not be your best option. You can reduce the impact on your joints by improving your technique.

Running can be a great complement to the body weight exercises incorporated within this program. If you are new to running or have not run much recently, start out slowly. Spend some time working on your form and gradually increase your pace and distance.

Depending on where you live, a treadmill may represent an excellent alternative to walking or running outdoors. Using a treadmill provides a controlled environment: you can adjust the temperature of the room, your speed, and even the elevation (percent incline), all at the touch of a button. In addition, treadmills have a flexible deck, reducing the impact on your joints.

Cycling

Cycling has increased in popularity over the years, largely due to the number of different modes available. Be it on the road, in the mountains or at your local club, there is no shortage of options.

Cycling, being a non-weight bearing, non-impact activity is easier on the joints than say running. It also provides an excellent workout for the legs, particularly the quadriceps (front of the thigh), which are not utilized as much in running. For this reason, cycling represents an excellent cross-training option for those who like to run, helping to balance out your muscles and giving your joints a break.

Rowing

If you have read the forward to this book, then you know that rowing holds a special place in my heart. Rowing is an exceptional form of exercise for a number of reasons. For the amount of time spent in the activity, you will burn more calories per minute than any of the other movements mentioned here. It is also a non-impact activity that provides a great overall workout. In addition to the aforementioned benefits, another plus is the relative low cost of a quality rowing machine when compared to a quality treadmill or indoor cycle. In fact, dollar for dollar, a rower represents one of the best pieces of exercise equipment money can buy.

Swimming

Swimming has many positive aspects to it. It works all your major muscle groups and provides a great cardiovascular workout too. Water is a buoyant environment and therefore exercising in water can be very therapeutic. It provides a much-needed rest from the effects of gravity on our bodies and is an excellent **complement** to any activity program. It should not, however, be your sole form of exercise.

We do not live in a buoyant environment and exercise in water does not provide the necessary *stress* to maintain our bone mass. In fact, studies of elite swimmers have found them to be lacking bone mass, and therefore are at a high risk for osteoporosis.

If fat loss is one of your main fitness goals, once again swimming is not the best choice of exercises as your main activity. While swimming is an excellent calorie burner, body fat functions as an insulator and also aids in buoyancy. The human body is adaptable and when frequently submerged in water will tend to hold onto body fat rather than release it for energy.

So, go ahead and get wet, just make sure to add in your body weight exercises and at least one of the other activities mentioned above into the mix.

Alternative Movements

If you are pressed for time or the conditions are not ideal to do one of the activities listed above try any of these options: dance, jump rope, squat thrusts (burpees), jumping jacks, or any other combination of body weight exercises. The key here is *movement* so go ahead, put on some music and get your groove on.

Monitoring Your Intensity

Among the variables discussed in **CHAPTER 2**, **FITT PRINCIPLES**, intensity is one the most important, yet least understood components. By understanding how the intensity level of your activity session affects your body's adaptation process you will be able to reach new heights with regard to your fitness level.

Before we get into some specific recommendations with regard to how hard to work, here are two common ways to measure your intensity:

> **Heart Rate** – Measured in bpm (beats per minute) using the formula: 208 – 0.7 X age = PMHR (Predicted Maximum Heart Rate). The predicted maximal heart rate is then multiplied by the desired exercise intensity, generally between 55 – 85% of your PMHR. The exact percentage is based on the individual's current fitness level and any health concerns they may have. Seek the assistance of a fitness professional for additional guidance.

This formula does not work for everyone. A percentage of the population has hearts that beat a bit faster or slower than average. For a more accurate assessment of your maximum heart rate have a stress test performed by a qualified professional.

Here are some examples for calculating the PMHR (Predicted Maximum Heart Rate) for a 30 and 55-year-old person, and then applying their PMHR to the ranges based on the formula described above:

PMHR: 208 – 0.7 X 30 (age) = 187
0.55 X 187 = bpm, 0.85 X 187 = bpm
Range: 103 – 159 bpm

PMHR: 208 – 0.7 X 55 (age) = 169
0.55 X 169 = bpm, 0.85 X 169 = bpm
Range: 93 – 144 bpm

A functional tool for measuring your level of intensity during your sessions is a heart rate monitor. The leading brand in heart rate monitors, **Polar** offers a wide variety of models. To learn more about Polar heart monitors visit my website, www.smartfittness.com

Ratings of Perceived Exertion (Effort) – Different scales are used to rate perceived exertion. For our purposes, we will use a 0 to 10 scale with 0 signifying no effort at all (seated or lying down), 6 illustrating a moderate intensity level, and 10 representing a maximum or all-out effort.

The following table is a modified Borg scale:

SCALE	EFFORT LEVEL/PHYSICAL SIGNS
0	No effort, seated or lying down
1	Beginning to move slowly
2	Increasing the pace slightly
3	Moving a bit faster still
4	Breathing rate noticeably increased
5	Breathing a bit heavier
6	Moderate effort, can pass the "talk test"
7	Slight burning sensation in muscles
8	Unpleasantly fatigued
9	Breathing deeply, muscles burning
10	Maximum effort – must stop

These physical signs will help you identify your intensity level:

. Your respiratory (breathing) rate – Pay attention to your breathing as you exercise. The "talk test" will help you identify if you are within your aerobic range. You should be able to carry on a conversation with someone without gasping for air or pausing to get your words out.

- Burning sensation in your muscles – Your muscles should feel warm during your sessions or you may even experience a slight burning sensation. If, however, it feels like someone set your muscles on fire, it's a good sign you are outside of your aerobic range. This burning sensation will typically be accompanied by the heavy breathing described above.

The use of heart rate and perceived exertion need not be mutually exclusive. By combining the two, you can compare the objective feedback your heart rate represents with the subjective sensations you are feeling. With practice, you will develop a keen sense of how hard you are working and can adjust your intensity accordingly.

Optimal Intensity Levels

Keep in mind; this program is not about going from a couch potato to Superman or Wonder Woman overnight. It is about **progressive adaptation**. Your body is capable of amazing things, however vast improvements in your fitness level happening overnight is not one of them. Here are some recommendations on where to start based on your current condition:

If you have been **primarily sedentary** for the past few months or longer, start slowly. In the first two to four weeks, go for a sensation of being *pleasantly fatigued* (HR 55 – 65% of Max or an RPE of 5 – 6) during your sessions. Due to your sedentary lifestyle, any physical demands placed on your body will be enough to stimulate the adaptive response. Give your body a chance to get used to the movements and the added stress to your system. Focus on your breathing and the way your body feels as you exercise. As your body adapts and you begin to get stronger **gradually** increase the intensity.

Once you have established a base level of fitness or if you are already **moderately active,** push yourself a little harder. Work at an intensity that is *slightly unpleasant* to *unpleasant* (HR 60 – 85% of Max or RPE of 6 – 8). As you continue exercising your tolerance for this discomfort will improve. You may even start to "love the burn" as many regular exercisers do.

When you have been **active consistently**, at least 8 to 12 weeks, try some high intensity sessions. During a high intensity session, you should approach or possibly reach exhaustion the point where, although you feel like you cannot continue, you push yourself until you are physically unable to go on. Your heart rate will approach or even reach its maximum (90 – 100% or an RPE of 9 – 10).

Caution – this level is only recommended for those with no known disease or physical restrictions. When in doubt, consult with your physician.

Do not work at a high intensity level too frequently. Depending on your recoverability and lifestyle, you may be able to work in one or two high intensity sessions per week, intermixed with some moderate or easy, active recovery days.

One of the best ways to improve your fitness level is via *Interval Training*. Interval Training involves increasing the intensity level for brief periods of time (intervals) within the session. You may have a *work* interval of 30 seconds to a minute followed by a *rest* interval of equal or greater amount of time. The length of each rest interval depends on these three interrelated factors:

1. How much higher the work interval is increased in comparison to your baseline pace. Example – If you go from an RPE of 5 to a work interval of 6 for one minute, you should then be able to recover within less than one minute (approximately 30 seconds). Conversely, you go from an RPE of 5 to a work interval of 8, and then you will likely need greater than one minute to recover.

2. How long the work interval lasts. Example – Your work interval is just 30 seconds long you should be able to recover within one minute or less. Rather if your work interval is 1 – 2 minutes, you may need an equal amount of time to recover.

3. Your fitness levels. As your fitness level improves, so will your ability to recover. Considering the examples above, instead of needing a minute to recover after the higher increase in your intensity, you will likely recover in 30 seconds or less.

The only way to find *your* optimal work/rest interval is through trial and error. In order to determine what works best, you need to keep records of each session.

Leisure Interest/Sport

In addition to the activities mentioned above, I encourage you to set goals for a leisure interest. This could be a sport such as golf, tennis or ultimate Frisbee or an event such as a community fun run or multi-sport event. It may also be something like hiking a particular trail or climbing a mountain you've had your eye on. The best choice is something challenging that you will enjoy working toward.

There is something special about the games we play or the activities we choose to unwind and relax. It's our passion for them that makes the activity that much more fun. If you do not already have a game or leisure interest that gets you excited, I highly recommend you find one.

CHAPTER 5
THE PROGRAM

<u>**Program Schedule**</u>

This program is designed to give you as much choice as possible while still maintaining the structure necessary to keep you on track and progressing. The more you enjoy the program, the more likely you are to do it regularly. In fact, the most important factor in regard to this program is that you do it on a daily or nearly daily basis.

I have set the first 28 days of the program to give you a foundation to work from. Following this period, I encourage you to mix up the movements to create variety within each session.

If you have an event such as a fun run, tennis tournament or some other activity coming up, you will need to adjust your schedule accordingly. You may eliminate one or two of your regular sessions and spend more time on skill practice specific to your event.

Should you find yourself missing more than a few sessions, get back into your routine as soon as possible. Don't let a few days off turn into a week, which before you know it turns into a month. The longer your break, the more difficult you will find getting back into a routine. Remember, consistency is key!

If you cannot do at least 8 consecutive repetitions of the following exercises, add this variation: Once you have completed as many reps as possible immediately begin an isometric contraction, holding a slightly flexed position for as long as you can. As your strength improves, you will be able to do more repetitions moving through the full range of motion.

Before you get started, remember, this program is intended for those who are apparently healthy with no known disease, joint or mobility problems. Before beginning this program, please see your doctor for a complete physical examination.

<u>**READY POSITION**</u>

Start each movement, unless otherwise noted from this position.

1. Stand tall, feet hip-width apart, chest out and shoulders back.

2. Relax your arms down by your sides and look straight ahead.

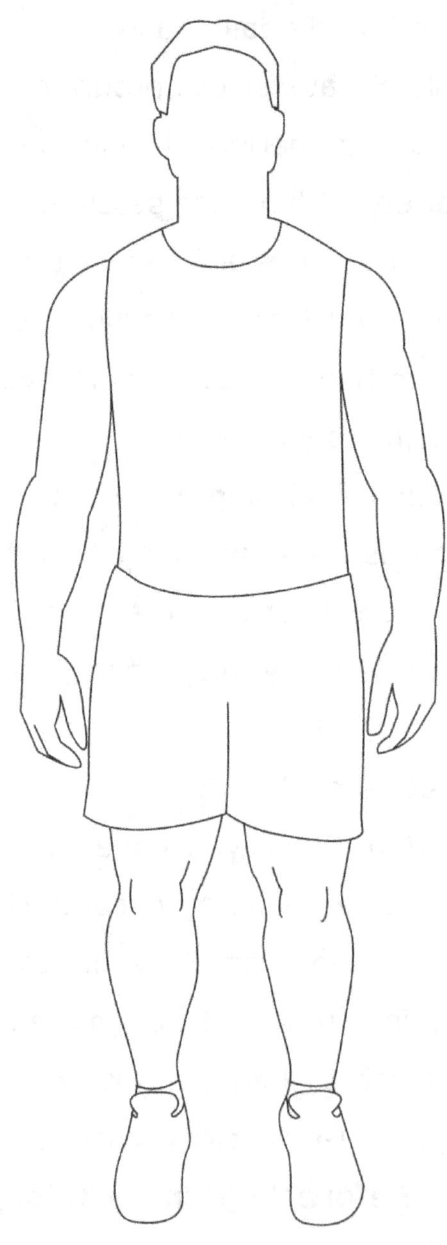

<u>**Warm-up**</u>

Here are three dynamic stretches to warm-up your muscles and prepare your body for more vigorous actions. Begin each session with these:

<u>**WINDMILL – SHOULDER ROTATIONS**</u>

A great way to begin your warm-up by getting your shoulders, chest and back loosened up.

1. Begin in the Ready Position.
2. Take a deep breath and raise both hands over head.
3. Exhale as you lower your right hand in front of you while simultaneously dropping your left hand behind you, circling around with both hands meeting overhead.
4. Continue breathing deeply as you rotate two times one direction and then reverse two times in the opposite direction.
5. Repeat three times each direction, then four times and then finally five times each direction.

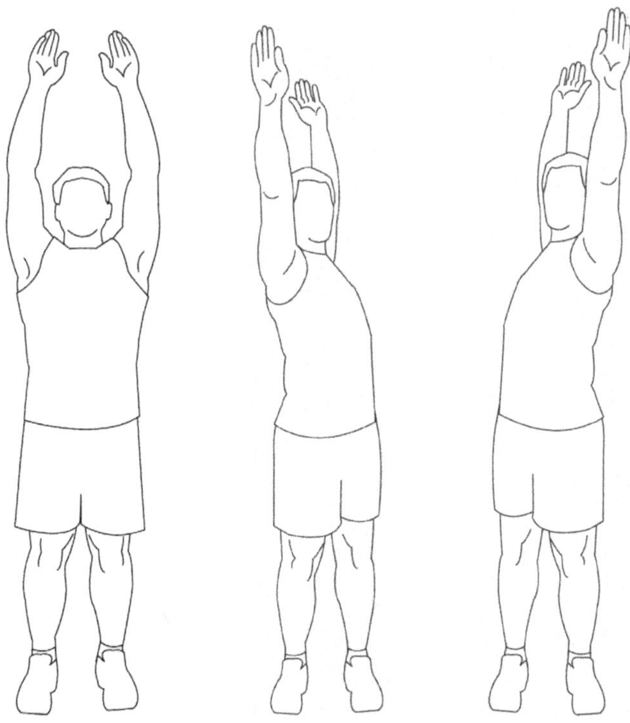

<u>**WAIST TURNER**</u>

An excellent overall body movement focusing on the torso:

1. Begin in the ready position.
2. Slowly begin to rotate to your left and then right back and forth.
3. Gradually increase your speed of rotation letting the momentum carry your arms around with you.
4. Let your hands gently slap your lower back and kidney area as you turn from side to side.
5. Breathe deeply as you rotate.
6. Repeat as desired, at least 20 times each direction.

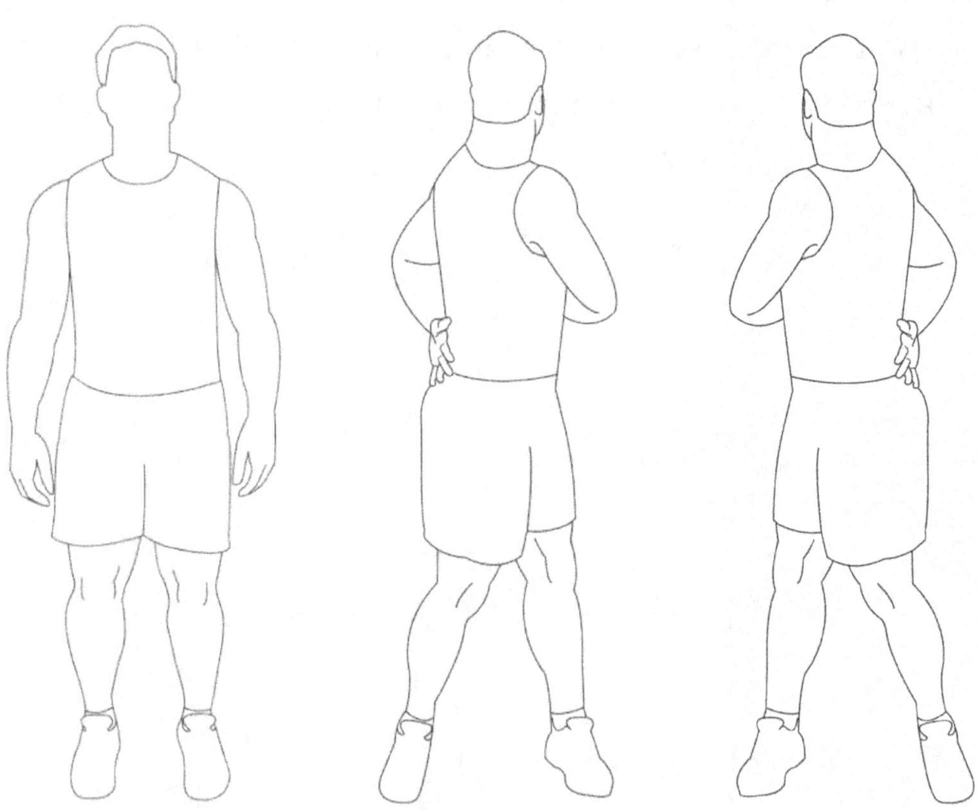

<u>**HIP CIRCLES**</u>

This one will loosen up your hips and thighs while also bringing your knees and ankles into the act.

1. From the ready position place your hands on your hips.
2. Bend your knees slightly and push your hips out and around in a circle like you are doing a hula dance (no grass skirt required).
3. Breathe freely as you rotate your hips twice around to the left then reverse around to the right.
4. Rotate each direction three times, and then four times and finally five times.

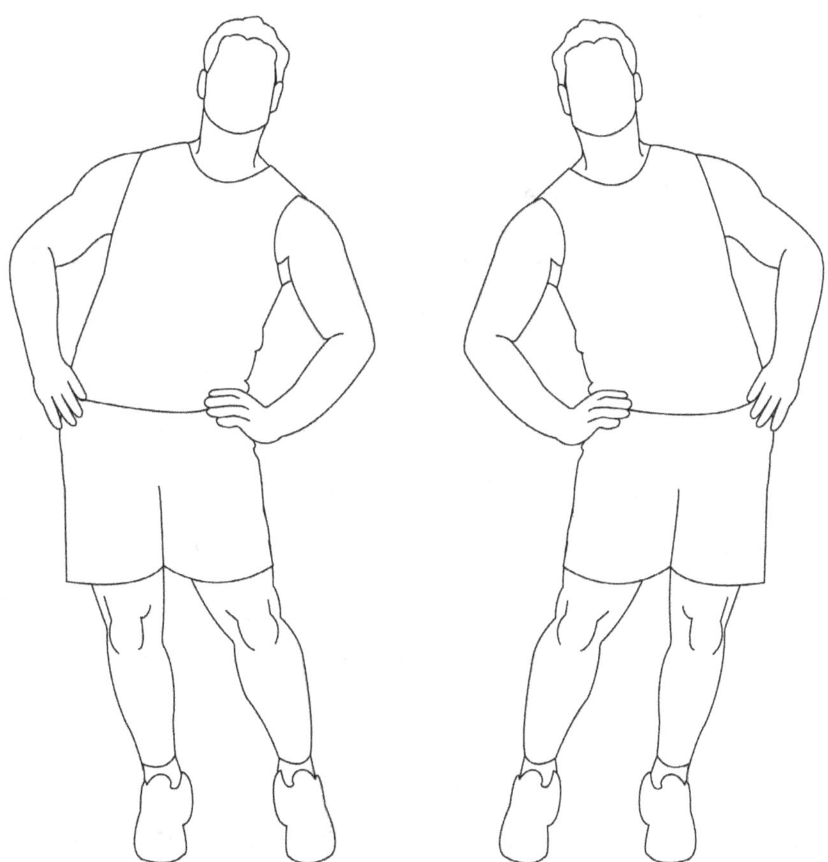

Day 1

CHAIR SQUAT

Sitting down and standing up are so commonplace that we take the actions for granted. Yet this *simple* act is not so simple after all. Consider that over 200 muscles are involved when squatting, requiring strength, balance and coordination.

Sitting down and standing up are so commonplace that we take the actions for granted. Yet this *simple* act is not so simple after all. Consider that over 200 muscles are involved when squatting, requiring strength, balance and coordination.

Sitting down and standing up are so commonplace that we take the actions for granted. Yet this *simple* act is not so simple after all. Consider that over 200 muscles are involved when squatting, requiring strength, balance and coordination.

1. Begin in the ready position.
2. Inhale deeply as you lower your body as if sitting down in a chair, keep your chest up and allow your arms to rise in front of you for balance.
3. Continue to lower your body as low as possible while maintaining your balance (heels stay down).
4. Don't worry about how low you get in the beginning. As you get used to the movement and your legs get stronger, you will be able to squat lower. Aim for a position with your thighs parallel to the floor.
5. Exhale as you stand up, lowering your arms by your side.
6. Repeat this sequence, working up to at least 30 repetitions.

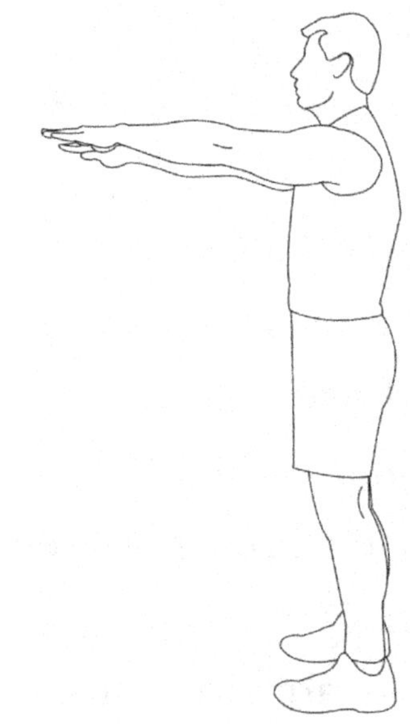

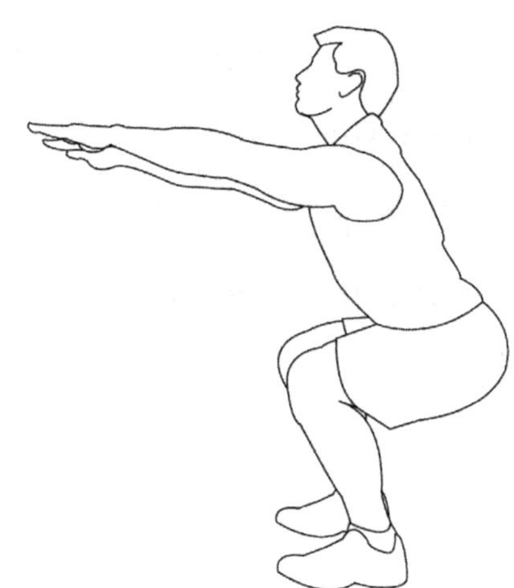

Day 1

<u>PUSHUP/MODIFIED PUSHUP</u>

Pushups are a fundamental exercise which develop your upper body strength, together with your torso and legs.

1. Place your hands on the floor slightly wider than shoulder-width apart and your feet (knees if modified) a few inches apart.
2. Begin with your arms extended and your body in a straight line.
3. Inhale as you lower your body until your chest is a few inches from the floor.
4. Keep the muscles in your torso and legs taut to stabilize your body. Move up and down as a single unit.
5. Push back up until your arms are straight.
6. Repeat as many times as you can, working up to at least 20 consecutive reps.

Note – The female is doing the full push-ups and the male the modified to illustrate a point. Some women may not need to modify their push-ups and some men might☺

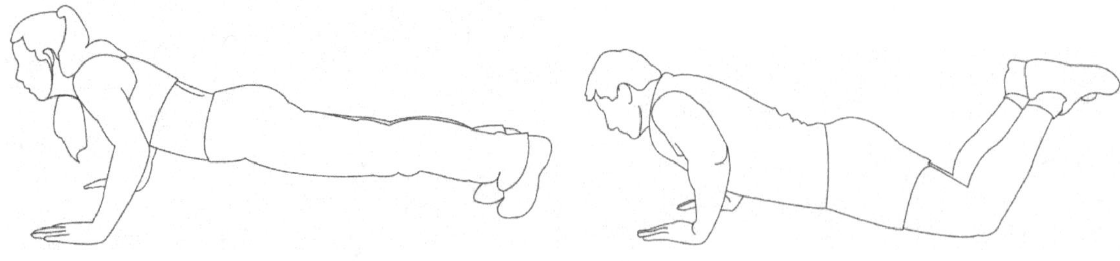

Day 1

<u>BENT-OVER ROW</u>

Here is a great exercise that focuses on your back, back of the shoulders and arms while using the rest of your muscles to stabilize your body position.

1. Begin in the ready position.
2. Inhale deeply as you squat down to pick up the weight.
3. Raise your upper body slightly, keeping your head and chest up to maintain a flat back.
4. Exhale as you pull your shoulders and elbows up toward the ceiling, raising the weight as high as you can.
5. Inhale as you lower the weight back down to a straight arm position, maintaining a flat back (head up and chest out) throughout the exercise.
6. Raise and lower the weight as many times as you can while maintaining your form. Aim for between 8-15 reps or until fatigued.
7. Once you have completed the set, lower the weight to the floor.

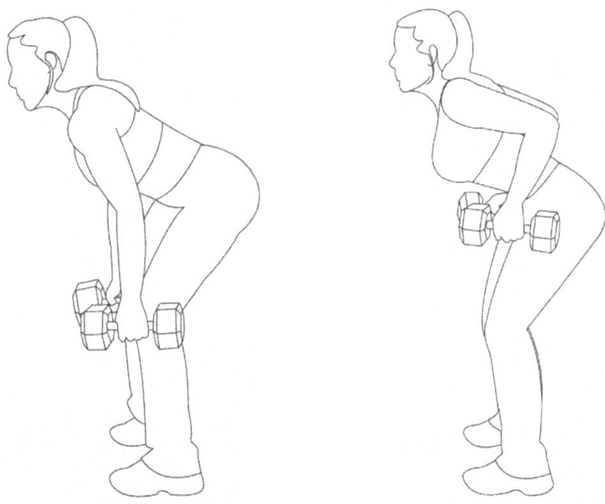

Day 2

<u>A to B with a PURPOSE</u>

Walk, jog, run, cycle, row or swim on this day. Remember to record your session in the *A to B with a Purpose Recording Form* found in Appendix B.

Day 3

<u>SQUAT & LIFT (DEAD LIFT)</u>

The squat & lift, also known as a dead lift, is a functional exercise designed to get ready for any lifting you may need to do in your everyday life. Learning this movement will help you avoid a back injury while also improving your body's overall condition.

1. From the ready position inhale deeply as you squat down and grab the weight in front of you.
2. Keep your head up and chest out as you pick up the weight, exhaling as you stand up.
3. Inhale as you slowly lower the weight back down to the floor.
4. Repeat between 6-12 reps with good form. If you cannot complete at least 6 reps, decrease the weight. If you can do more than 12 reps without fatigue, increase the weight.

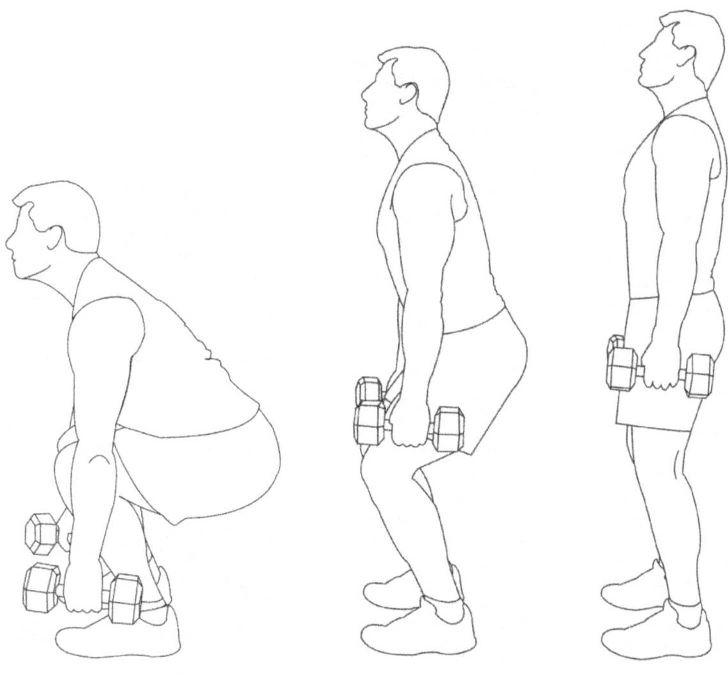

Day 3

STANDING SHOULDER PRESS

Everyday life occasionally requires us to lift something heavy overhead, placing something on a shelf for example. This exercise will help prepare you for such an occasion.

1. Begin in the ready position.
2. Inhale as you squat down and grab the weight.
3. Keep your head up and chest out as you stand up with the weight, exhaling as you stand up. (See squat and lift on previous page).
4. Inhale before you move and then exhale as you press the weight overhead.
5. Inhale as you lower the weight to shoulder level.
6. Repeat pressing the weight overhead, between 6-12 reps with good form. If you cannot complete at least 6 reps, decrease the weight. If you can do more than 12 reps without feeling fatigued, increase the weight.

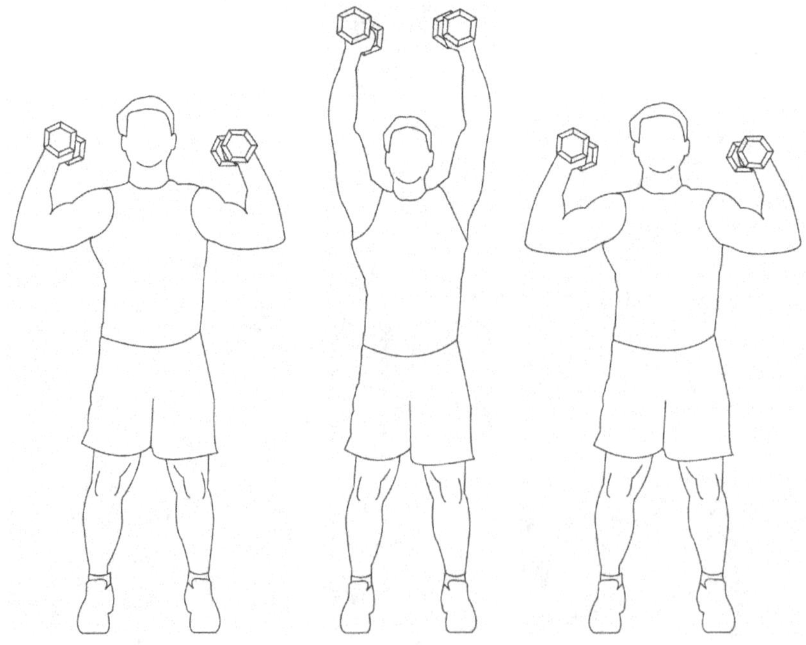

Day 3

<u>TORSO BOW & ARC</u>

Here is a dynamic way to work your torso, strengthening and stretching your abdominals and back muscles.

1. Begin in the ready position.

2. Exhale and flex forward slowly, contracting your abdominals, hold for a second or two fully flexed.

3. Extend backward as you inhale, hold for a couple seconds in extension, and then exhale as you return to center.

4. Repeat the sequence, gradually increasing how far you flex forward and extend back, as your muscles loosen up.

5. Repeat, forward and back at least 10 times.

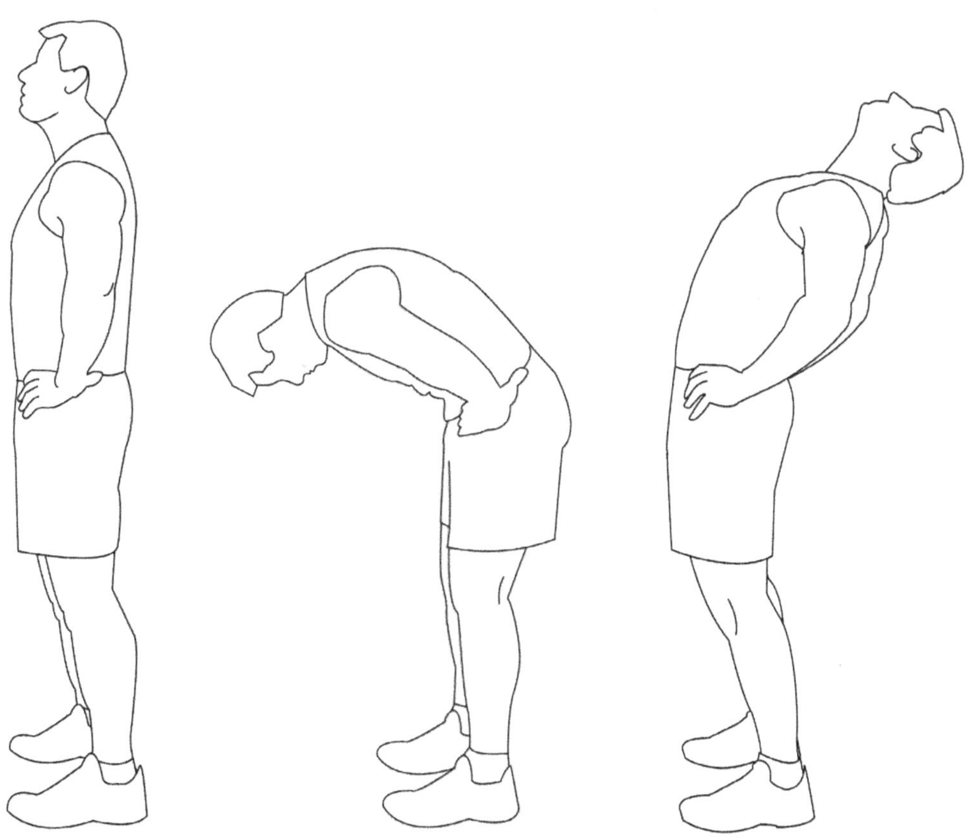

Day 4

A to B with a PURPOSE

Depending on what you did on Day 2, you may want to do the same activity or mix it up with one of the others. If you swam then I recommend you work in some weight bearing activity today. Whatever you end up doing, record your session in the *A to B with a Purpose Recording Form* found in Appendix B.

Day 5

SPLIT SQUATS

This movement will strengthen your legs and improve your balance. In addition, Split Squats are part of a progression for an upcoming exercise, lunges.

1. Begin in the ready position.
2. Step forward with your left leg about twice your normal stride while maintaining a shoulder width apart stance.
3. Inhale deeply as you lower your body down. Keep your chest up and your back straight.
4. Continue to lower your body until your front and back legs form 90-degree angles at the knees. Your front foot's heel will remain on the ground; however, you will raise the heel on your back foot.
5. Exhale as you straighten your legs to raise your body up but remain in the over-stride (lunge) position.
6. Repeat flexing and extending your legs aiming for at least 10 reps.
7. Change legs and repeat as above.

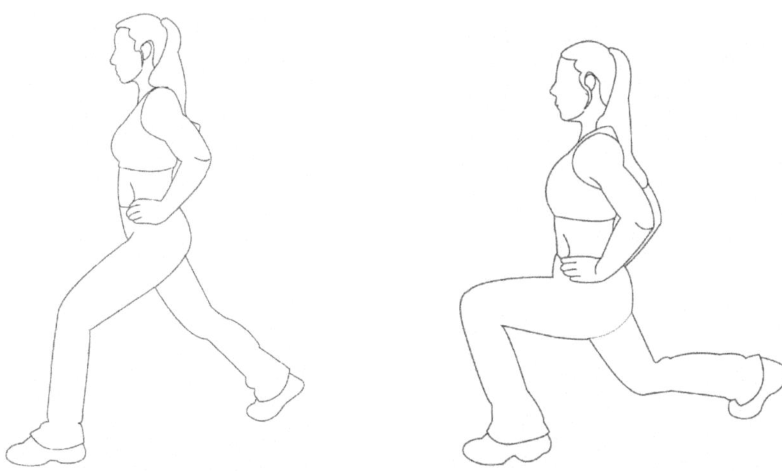

Day 5

MODIFITED V-UP/V-UP

V-ups provide a dynamic way to work your torso while getting your whole body into the act.

1. Start out flat on your back with your arms stretched out over your head.

2. Raise your hands and knees or feet together, meeting at the top. The timing and coordination of this exercise takes some practice. In time you will find your hands and feet coming together in the desired "V" position.

3. If you find these difficult to complete more than a couple of reps modify the movement this way: Bend your legs and draw your knees toward your chest and your arms come forward reaching toward your feet.

4. Repeat the V-up, modified V-up or a combination of both working up to at least 20 reps.

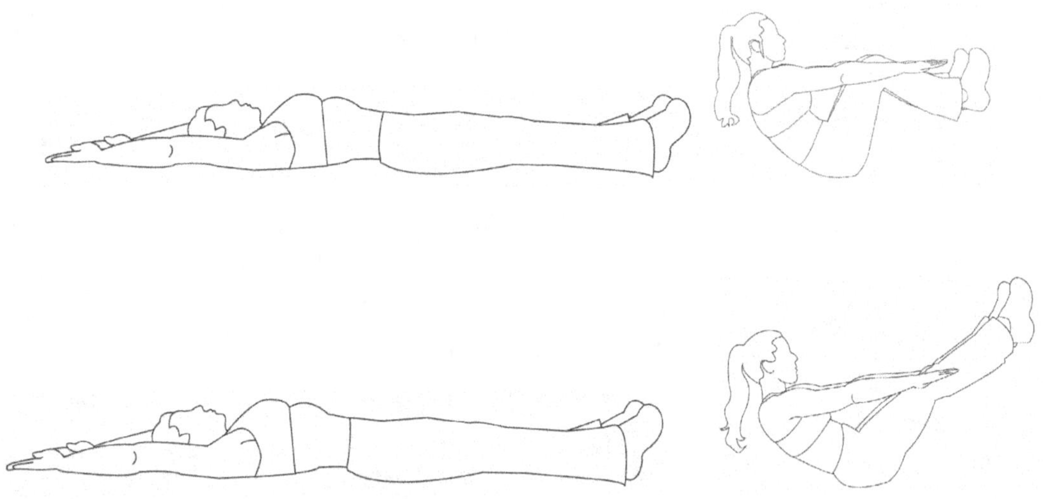

Day 5

<u>BACK EXTENSIONS</u>

Back Extensions are important in strengthening the torso and creating balance between your abdominals and the erector muscles of the lower back.

1. Begin on your stomach lying face down with your arms by your side.

2. Inhale and then exhale as you extend your back, raising your head, neck, chest and abdomen off the floor. Simultaneously press your hands toward the ceiling as you arch upward.

3. Your legs and feet remain on the ground.

4. Lower your body back down slowly until your chin touches the floor.

5. Repeat until fatigued, working up to at least 20 reps.

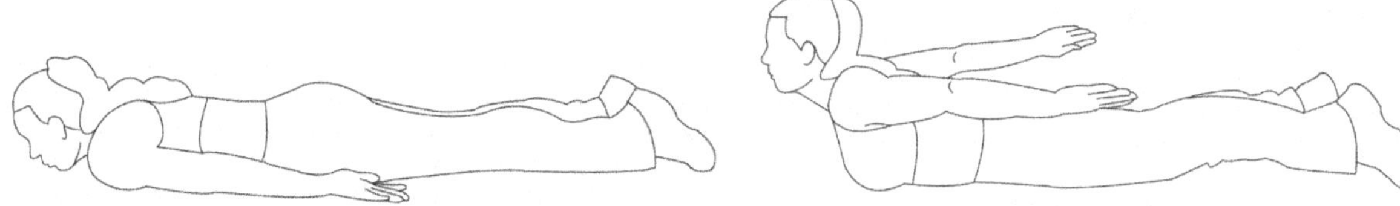

Day 6

<u>A to B with a PURPOSE</u>

You are approaching the end of your first week on the program. You may be feeling a bit fatigued today depending on how well you have slept and fed your body the past few days/nights. Adjust your intensity and time accordingly as you walk, jog, run, cycle, row or swim today. As always, record your session in the *A to B with a Purpose Recording Form* found in Appendix B.

Day 7

<u>ACTIVE RECOVERY</u>

This is a day for you to relax a bit and recover from the previous six days of activity. Rest, however, does not mean turning into a couch potato. Your body will recover optimally through some light activity. Go for a relaxing walk, stretch, dance, anything really. Just move your body and have fun!

Days 8 – 14

Continue your program by repeating the previous seven days of activity, adding a second set of each movement and going a bit further or faster on your A to B days. Do not sacrifice your form to increase your numbers; rather stay focused on keeping your movements smooth and your body in alignment. As your body adapts over the weeks ahead you will be amazed at what you can do.

Day 15

CHAIR SQUAT ISO-HOLD

Remember wall-sits from P.E.? If you don't, this exercise is sure to refresh your memory. If you have not done these before, well then you are in for a *treat*. Do not overdo this exercise; otherwise, you will find walking and sitting down difficult in the days that follow.

1. Begin in the ready position.

2. Inhale deeply as you lower your body as if sitting down in a chair, keep your chest up and allow your arms to rise in front of you for balance. If you find it difficult to maintain your balance, you may lean against a wall.

3. Continue to lower your body until your thighs are parallel to the floor (heels stay down).

4. Hold this position as you breathe into the squat. Aim for 15 to 30 seconds for starters, gradually working up to sets of at least one minute.

5. Stand up, lowering your arms by your side.

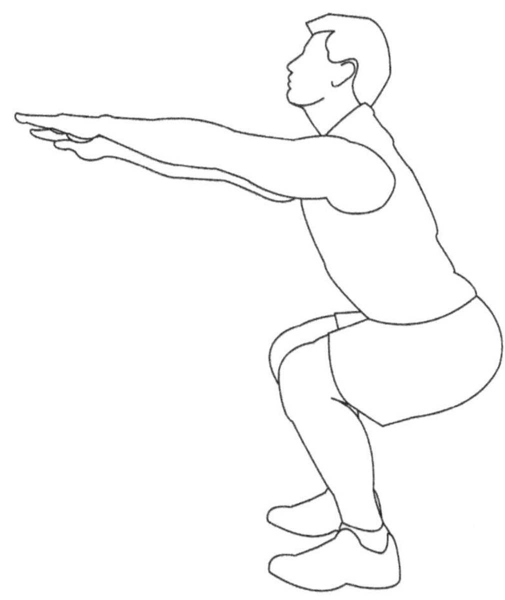

Day 15

PUSH-UP/MODIFIED PUSH-UP ISO-HOLD

This is a great way to further develop your strength throughout the entire body and will also help you increase your numbers on pushups.

1. Place your hands on the floor slightly wider than shoulder-width apart and your feet (knees if modified) a few inches apart.
2. Begin with your arms extended and your body in a straight line.
3. Bend your arms slightly and then hold this position.
4. Keep the muscles in your torso and legs taunt to stabilize your body.
5. Breathe deeply as you continue to maintain a flat body. Go for 15 to 30 seconds for to start, gradually working up to sets of at least one minute.
6. You may vary the amount of flexion in through your shoulders and elbows to alter the effect.

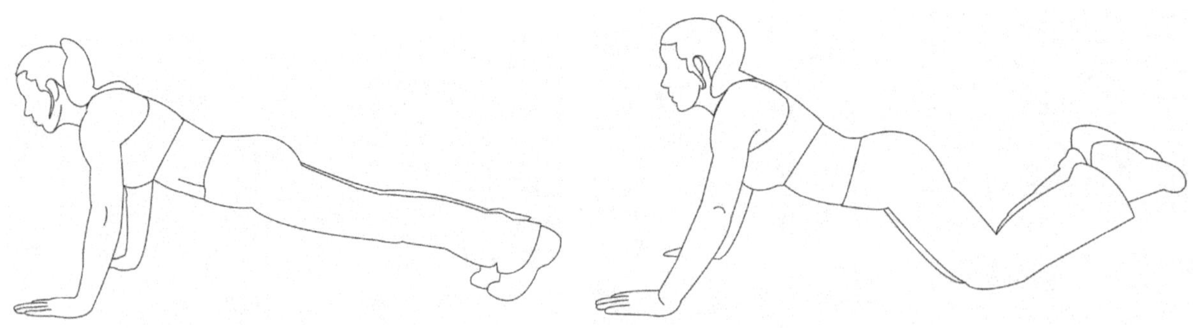

Day 15

<u>SEATED ROW ISO-HOLD</u>

Here is another iso-hold that will increase your strength and stabilization through your back, shoulders and arms. This exercise requires the use of a *Yoga Strap*.

1. Begin seated on the floor with your legs out in front of you slightly bent.
2. Grab the strap near either end and wrap it around the middle of your feet.
3. Be sure you have a good grip on the strap and then slide it around until you have equal lengths on either side (hands side by side).
4. Sit up tall and begin pulling your shoulders and elbows back.
5. Breathe into this iso-hold keep your chin up and your chest up and out. Maintain this position as you continue pulling.
6. Hold this position and breathe deeply for at least 15-30 seconds, working up to 1 minute or longer.
7. Ease out of the hold and release the strap.

If you do not have a strap lie down on your back with your arms by your sides at a 90-degree angle drive the back of your upper arms into the floor.

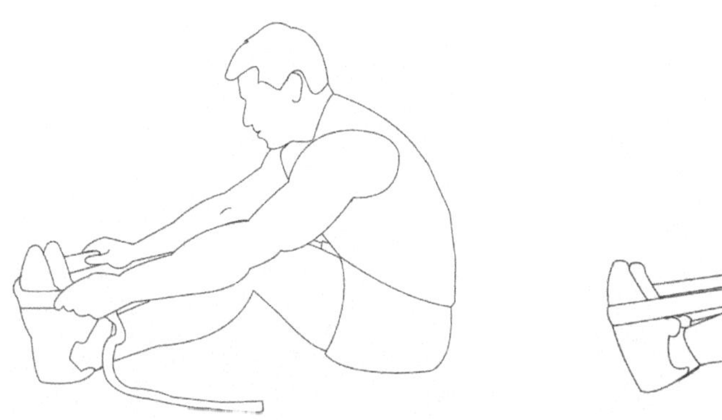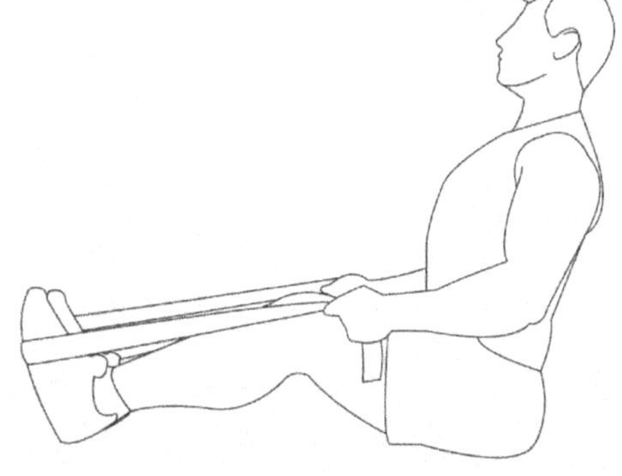

Day 16

A to B with a PURPOSE

These next two weeks, starting today, begin to increase the intensity level or duration of your activity. Today, go a little bit harder by working in some intervals. If you need a refresher on this concept and how to monitor your intensity levels review that section within chapter 4. Continue to record your sessions in the *A to B with a Purpose Recording Form* found in Appendix B.

Day 17

<u>LUNGE/WALKING LUNGE</u>

This movement will strengthen your legs and improve your balance in similar but more dynamic fashion than the split squats that you preformed earlier.

1. Begin in the ready position.

2. Inhale as you step (lunge) forward with your right leg about twice your normal stride while maintaining a shoulder width apart stance.

3. Lower your body until your front and back legs form 90-degree angles at the knees. Your front foot's heel will remain on the ground, but you will raise the heel on your back foot.

4. Exhale as you push back to a standing position, maintaining a shoulder-width stance.

5. Now step out with your left leg in the same manner as above and push back to a standing position. Repeat, alternating legs and aiming for at least 10 reps on each side.

6. To increase the intensity of this exercise, repeat the movement on the same leg for the desired number of repetitions before switching legs.

7. For walking lunges follow steps 1 through 3, but then instead of pushing back to a standing position, stand up over that front leg. Now lunge out with the opposite leg, walking along in a lunge position.

8. Continue the walking lunges until you have completed 10 reps on each leg.

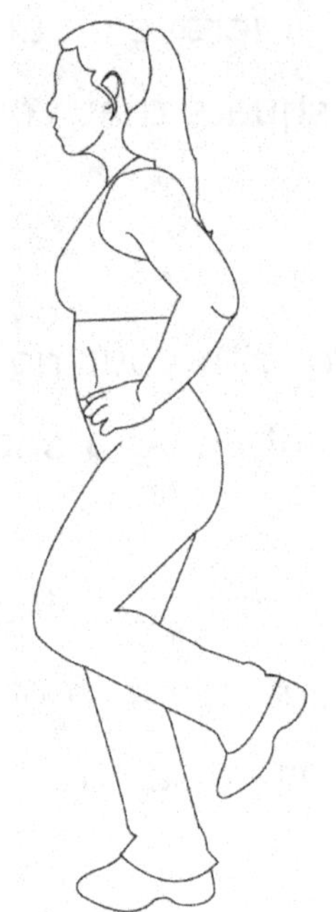

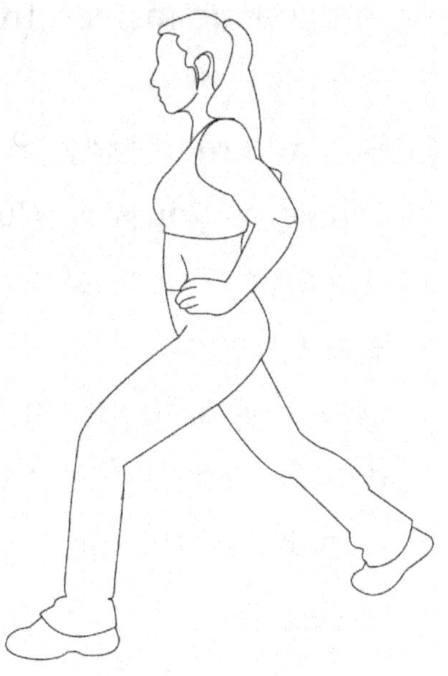

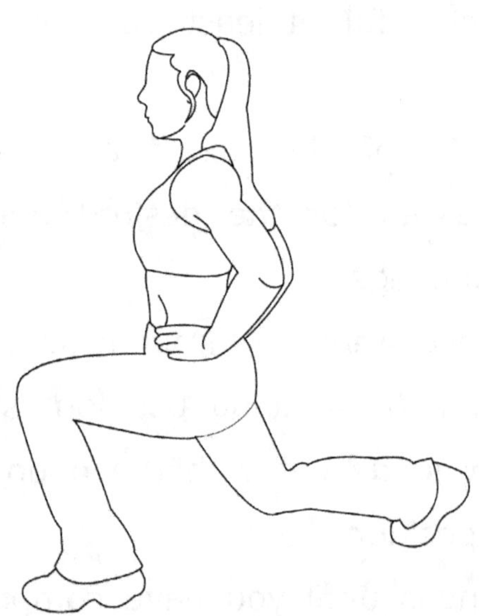

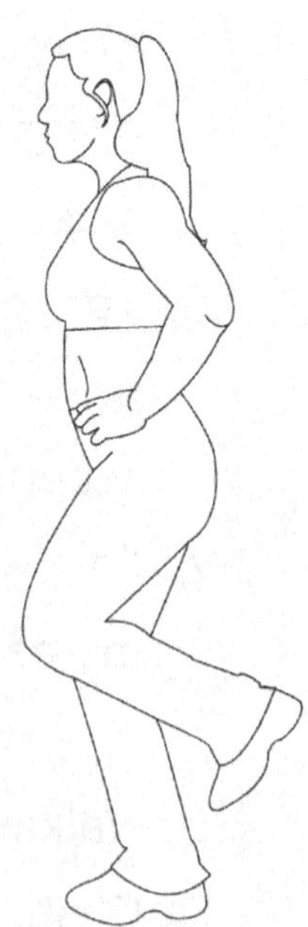

Day 17

<u>PLANK</u>

This isometric exercise will increase your strength and stabilization, throughout your whole body.

1. Begin lying face down and bend your arms at a 90-degree angle, elbows under your shoulders and your feet a few inches apart.
2. Extend your body so that you are supported on your forearms and feet, maintaining a straight line with your body.
3. Don't let your hips drop, focusing on contracting the muscles in your torso, butt and legs.
4. Hold this position, breathing deeply for 10-30 seconds.
5. Ease out of the position by lowering your body to the floor.
6. As a variation, plank off of your hands like in a pushup position.

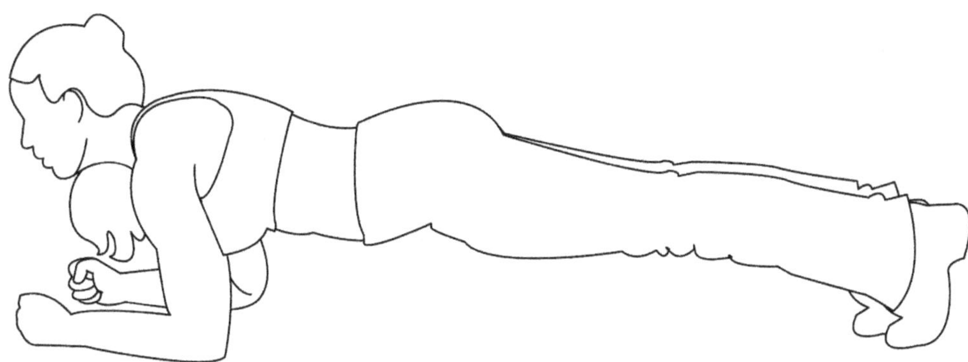

Day 17

<u>BACK EXTENSION ISO-HOLD</u>

Improve the strength and stability of your torso by creating balance between your abdominals and low back muscles (erector spinae).

1. Begin on your stomach lying face down with your arms by your side.
2. Inhale and then exhale as you extend your back raising your head, neck, chest and abdomen off the floor. Simultaneously press your hands toward the ceiling as you arch upward.
3. Your legs and feet remain on the ground.
4. Hold this position, breathing deeply for 10-30 seconds.
5. To increase the difficulty of this exercise, extend your arms overhead.

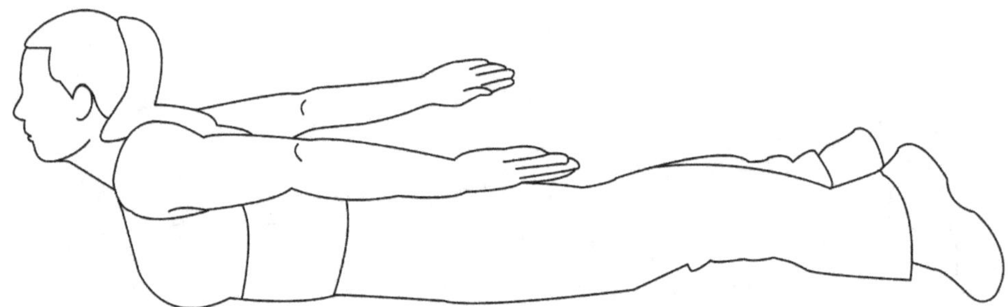

Day 18

A to B with a PURPOSE

By now you will have built up your endurance and feel like you can go a little bit longer during your sessions. If time permits, today would be a good day to increase the duration of your activity by 5 to 10 minutes. You will need to keep your intensity moderate as you go a bit longer, working primarily on endurance this session. Continue to record your sessions in the *A to B with a Purpose Recording Form* found in Appendix B.

Day nineteen begins on the next page. There are only two exercises on this day since these movements require greater practice and higher energy demands than some of the previous days. Because Indian wrestlers have used these exercises for hundreds of years, some sources refer to the exercises as Hindu Squats and Hindu Pushups. I have changed the names of the exercises to Deep Squats and Arcing Pushups, descriptive names of the movements themselves.

Day 19

DEEP SQUAT

This exercise will strengthen your lower body while also giving you a fantastic cardiovascular workout. Do this movement a bit faster than the previous exercise in this program. As a reference, you should be able to do 25-30 consecutive repetitions in 45 seconds, 50 reps in about 75 to 90 seconds or 100 reps in 2 ½ to 3 minutes.

1. Begin in the ready position.
2. Inhale as you draw your hands in toward your chest.
3. Lower your body straight down, keeping your back as straight as possible.
4. As you squat down your hands fall back behind you and then down toward the floor.
5. Lower your body to a full squat with your thighs parallel to the floor and heals rising up off the floor.
6. Exhale as you swing your arms out in front, pushing off your toes to a standing position.
7. Repeat as desired, working up to at least 50 consecutive reps.

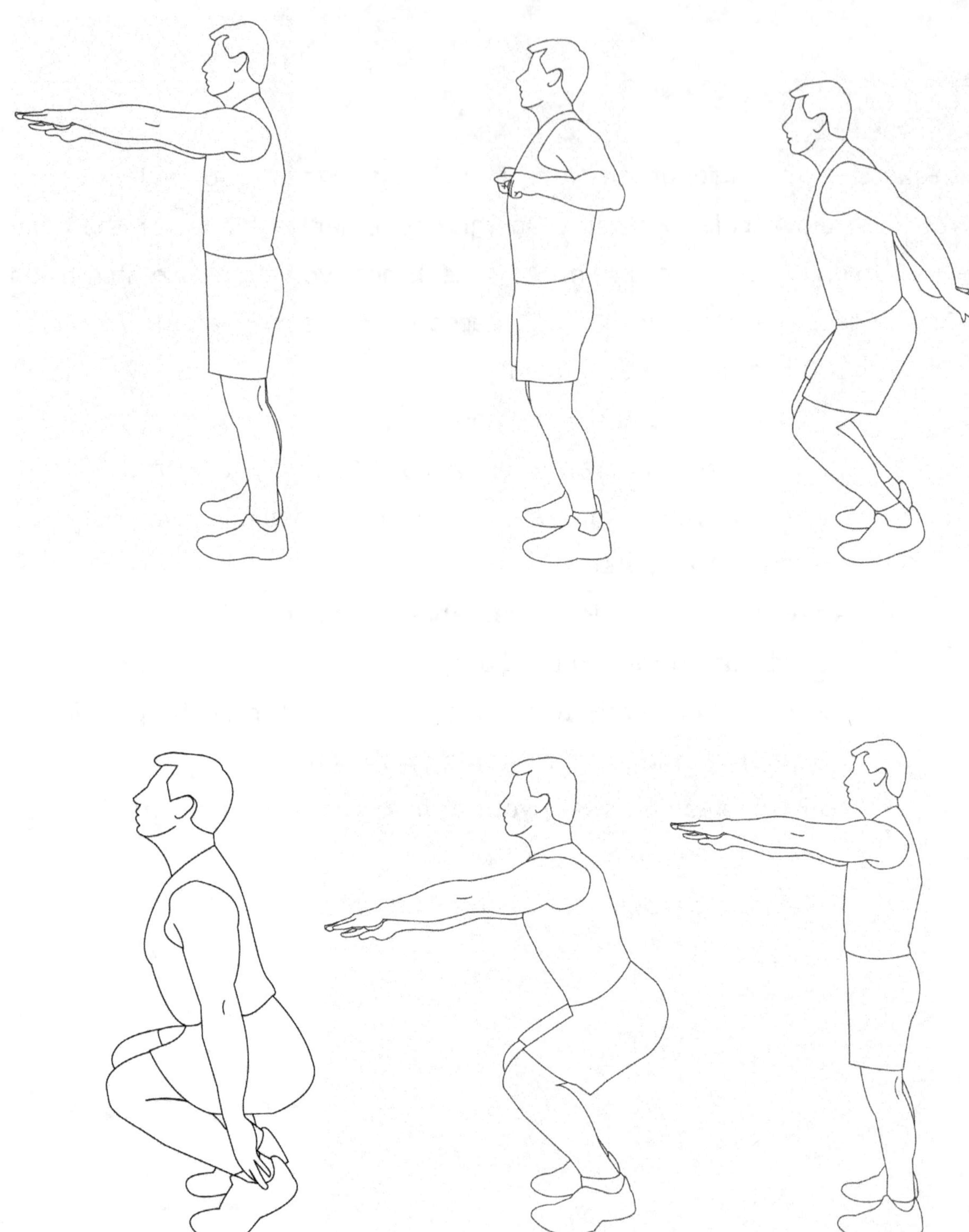

Day 19

<u>ARCING PUSH-UP</u>

A dynamic way to work your whole body: while you will gain greater strength/endurance throughout your upper body, you will also increase your flexibility in your shoulders, back and hips. Due to the large amount of muscle used through a large range of motion, you will also achieve a great cardiovascular workout.

1. Place your hands on the floor slightly wider than shoulder-width apart and your feet slightly wider than hip-width apart.
2. Start with your butt in the air, head between your arms, looking back at your feet.
3. Inhale and then begin to exhale as you bend your arms and lower your body in an arc, leading with your head, then chest, abdomen, hips and thighs, all barely off the ground as you come through.
4. Extend your arms and arch your back as you look up toward the ceiling, stretching through the hips, shoulders and back.
5. Keeping your arms straight raise your hips and push back toward your feet. Inhaling as you return to the starting position.
6. Repeat this sequence for as many reps as you can, working up to at least 25 consecutive repetitions.
7. If you get tired, **do not** drop to your knees, rather stay in the starting position, breathe and recover until you can continue, completing as many repetitions as you can.

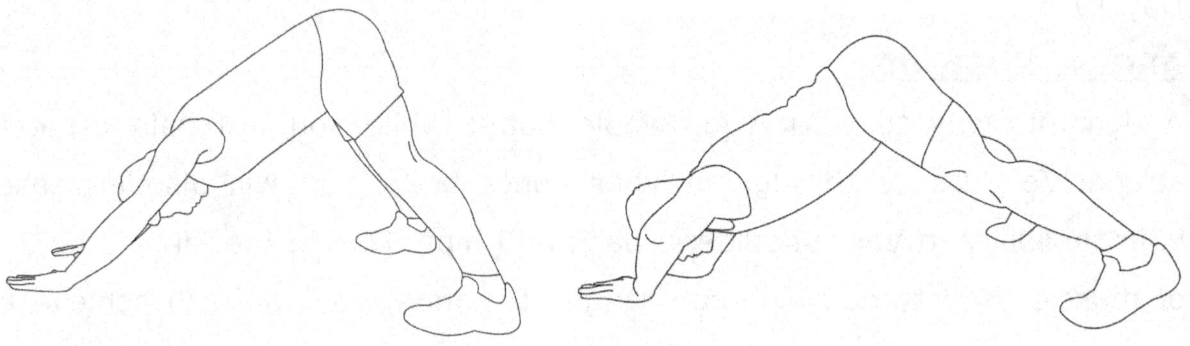

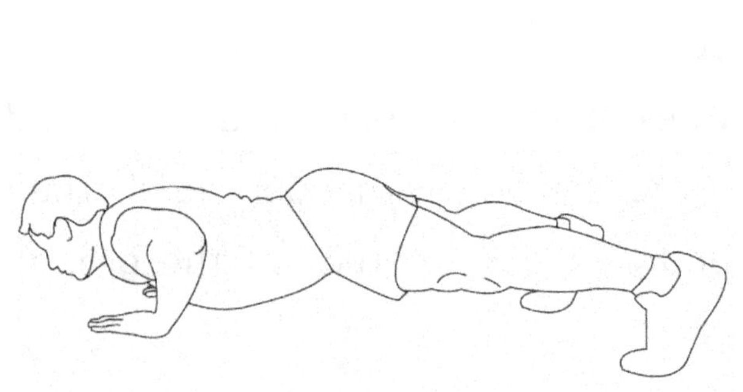

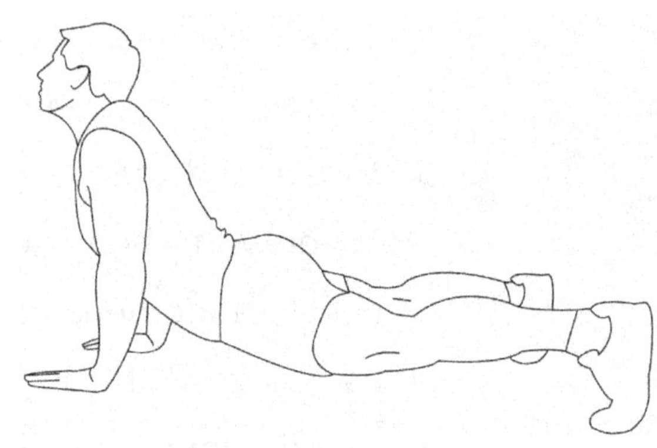

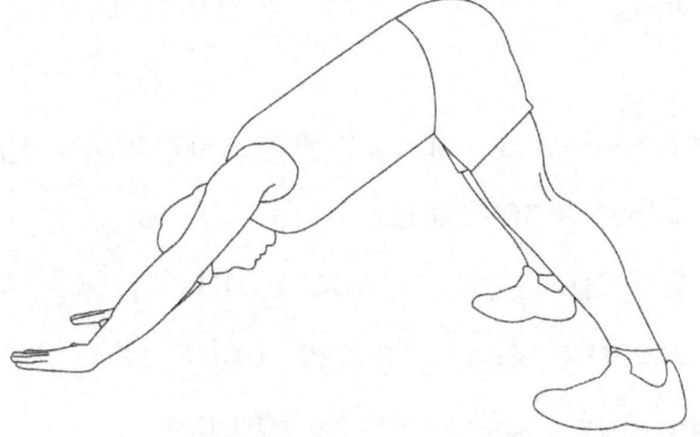

Day 20
A to B with a PURPOSE

You are approaching the end of your third week on the program and may be feeling a bit fatigued today. If you are moderately fatigued, or just flat out tired, listen to your body. Adjust your intensity and duration of your activity to match your state of recovery. Stay positive and focus on having fun as you walk, jog, run, cycle or swim today. Record your session in the *A to B with a Purpose Recording Form*.

Day 21
<u>ACTIVE RECOVERY</u>

Having pushed your body through another active week it is time to focus on recovery. You may choose from a variety of relaxing activities; a leisurely walk, some passive stretching, or even a dry sauna and massage to help release some tension.

Days 22 – 28

Continue your program by repeating the previous seven days of activity, adding a second or third set of each movement and going a bit further or faster on your A to B days. Do not sacrifice your form to increase your numbers, rather stay focused on keeping your movements smooth and your body in alignment. As your body adapts over the weeks ahead, you will be amazed at what you can do.

CHAPTER 6
TEN KEYS TO FUELING YOUR BODY RIGHT

As the saying goes, "We are what we eat." Since our body's cells are continually dying off and new ones are being formed every second, this saying couldn't be more true. Unfortunately, in our fast paced, fast food societies, the building blocks we often provide for our body's repair process are not ideal.

Applying the following nutritional principles will make a huge difference when it comes to your health. Changing your eating habits takes time, so be patient, yet persistent during this process as the rewards of optimal health and vitality will be well worth it.

Ten Keys to Fueling Your Body Right

1. Understand the difference between hunger and appetite. Hunger is physiological, while appetite is psychological. Hunger is the *need* for food, appetite is the *desire* for food. I am not implying that you shouldn't enjoy your food. Healthy foods taste good. Just eat primarily to satisfy hunger, not appetite.

2. When you are hungry, satisfy your hunger with nutrient dense foods. Nutrient dense foods contain a large number of vitamins, minerals, fiber, and phytochemicals compared to a relatively small number of calories. Eating nutrient dense foods satisfies. Vegetables, especially dark green leafy vegetables represent the best example of nutrient dense foods. Other good examples of nutrient dense foods include: fruit, seafood, and lean meats.

3. Avoid over-eating by eating food as close to its natural state as possible. If the food comes in a box, bag, or wrapper and has a long list of ingredients then it should be eaten in moderation if at all.

When the quality of the food you eat improves, the quantity of food you eat will automatically decrease. Healthy foods are naturally high in fiber and therefore more filling. When you focus on eating the right types of foods, portion control becomes less of an issue.

4. Minimize empty calories. Empty calories are food sources that contain a large number of calories but very little nutritional value. Empty calories are also quickly converted to sugar in our bloodstream, increasing the likelihood that these calories will be stored as fat. Examples of empty calories include: cakes, candy, pastries, chips, and sweet drinks such as soda. Consider how you can eat a whole bag of chips and still not be satisfied. You start thinking, okay that was good but what's next. When was the last time you were searching for something else to eat right after eating a nutrient dense meal of lean meat with stir-fried vegetables or a garden salad with tuna?

   As mentioned above, there is nothing wrong with enjoying a sweet treat now and then. The key is to enjoy that treat *after* a healthy meal or snack not instead of healthy food. By eating something nutrient dense first, you will be able to satisfy your sweet or salty craving with a small serving size afterward.

5. Increase the amount of healthy fats in your diet. Essential fatty acids, particularly omega-3 fatty acids are important for our cardiovascular system and also joint health. Rich sources of omega-3's include: cold-water fish like salmon, nuts & seeds such as walnuts, flax, and chia seeds.

6. Reduce the amount of unhealthy trans fats in your diet. Trans fats are found in deep fried foods common in fast food restaurants, and processed foods like chips, doughnuts, muffins, cakes and pie crusts.

7. Eat more fruits and vegetables. Still the biggest mistake most people make is not eating enough of these important foods. Fruits and vegetables are abundant in nature for a reason. They contain so many vital components, from life-promoting nutrients to lifesaving Phyto-chemicals which are linked to the prevention of many types of cancer. Include a multitude of colors for you fruit and vegetable intake, as the greater the variety, the more likely you are to take in all the essential components.

   Here are some suggestions to add more fruit and vegetables to your daily intake:

   - Fruit is a great way to start your day. Enjoy a small piece of fruit or a half-cup of berries for breakfast. Fruit also serves as a healthy snack or desert. Excellent fruits to include are: apricots, apples, kiwis, and cantaloupe. Some of the most nutrient dense berries are blueberries, blackberries, and strawberries.
   - Think of vegetables as the main course and your meat, poultry, seafood, eggs, or starch as the side dish. There are numerous ways to incorporate leafy greens into your eating plan: make a salad, use them as a wrap instead of a tortilla, add them to soup, steam them, or stir fry them with your favorite protein source. Aim for at least four servings of multi-colored, non-starchy vegetables every day. At least two of these servings should be

dark green leafy vegetables. Good choices of dark green leafy vegetables include: Swiss chard, kale, broccoli, turnip greens, collards, spinach, mustard greens, and lettuce (romaine, green and red leaf).

8. Reduce or eliminate the amount of alcohol you drink. Like most things, moderation is really the key here. Although studies have shown that 1 to 2 drinks per day will raise the levels of HDL's (good cholesterol), alcohol is a killer when it comes to packing on the weight. A glass of wine or shot of alcohol is 100+ calories (more for sweet liquors). In addition, having a drink with your meal can be a double whammy as alcohol negatively effects with the digestive process. If you enjoy a glass of wine or a beer with a meal now and then you'll be fine. Just make it a treat, not a nightly occurrence.

9. Stay Well Hydrated – Your body is comprised of between 60% to 70% water. The functions of water in your body are numerous, including but not limited to: temperature regulation, blood circulation, carrying nutrients and oxygen to cells and removing toxins and other waste products. In addition, a loss of just **3% of total body water will result in fatigue**.

   There has been some debate regarding how much water is enough. Some guidelines have been given as to how much water to drink in relation to your body weight. This however, does not take into account important factors such as individual activity levels, climate in which the activity is performed, and other dietary factors. As a general rule, drink one-half ounce per pound of body weight (divide your body weight by 2 to get your number of ounces per day). For example, someone who weighs 180 pounds would drink 90 ounces of water per day. If you work off the metric system divide your body weight in kilos by 30 to get an average amount in liters. For example, someone who weighs 80 kilos would drink 2.4 liters of water per day.

One of the best ways to ensure that you drink enough water each day is to drink on a regularly scheduled basis. Here is an example:

- Upon rising drink 8 to 12 ounces (400 to 600 ml.) of water.

- Re-hydrate following your workout. A good way to measure the amount of water lost during your workout is to weigh before and then after each session. For optimal recovery replace one to one and a half times the water weight lost during the activity. Fifteen fluid ounces of water equals one pound (500 milliliters equal half a kilo).

- Carry a water bottle so that you may drink some on the way to and coming home from school or work.

- Have a glass of water before you go to bed.

10. Supplement to fill in the gaps – Think of food supplements as nutritional insurance. Quality food supplements fill in the gaps from our less than perfect eating habits. Keep in mind the word supplement though. **Supplements should be a complement to, not a substitute for a balanced diet.** For years I have taken a quality multi-vitamin/mineral supplement. I also take vitamin D during the winter months, and fish oil since I do not consume foods rich in omega-3's on a daily basis. Consult with your healthcare provider for specific recommendations.

Remember, eating healthfully does not mean depriving oneself, as natural foods taste great. It is a matter of acquiring a taste for the natural flavors of whole food. It is likely your taste buds have become less sensitive due to the highly processed, sugar-laden foods that are common today. I promise, as you reduce and/or eliminate the fast food and junk food in your diet, you will become more aware of the natural flavors in whole foods.

CHAPTER 7

YOUR PLAN IN *ACTION*

AKA – YOUR REAR IN GEAR

<u>Getting Started</u>

There are two simple rules that are essential for success in anything:

1) Get Started – One of my favorite quotes I heard from a colleague recently is, "You don't have to be great to start, but you do have to start to be great." Starting is half the done. There will be days when you don't feel like doing your program. When this happens, review your goals and then get started. Surprisingly, some of these sessions will end up being your best.

2) Keep Going (persist) – Once you have started the program all you have to do is **keep doing it**. When it comes to maintaining our body's functionality the *law of use* applies: "**Use it or lose it**."

Here are six tips to help get you started and keep you going:

1. Wear loose, comfortable clothing that breathes. Cotton or other natural fibers are best. If you have a non-skid surface such as a rubber mat you do not need to wear shoes. Doing the exercises barefoot will strengthen your feet. If you are exercising on carpet, hardwood or any other slippery surface, wear a sport shoe that is not too stiff.

2. Invite a friend or family member to join you in your quest for greater fitness. You will be of great support to one another and the increased accountability will help you both stay on track.

3. Whenever possible, do your program in the morning. The earlier in the day you do your activity, the less likely something else will get in the way. In addition, morning sessions help boost your metabolism so that you will burn more calories throughout the day. Remember, if you are finding it difficult to schedule a block of time for your sessions, break them up into two or three mini-

sessions. The most important thing is that you do it, no matter what time of the day or night it gets done.

4. Do not exercise on a full stomach. Typically, you should wait 1 to 2 hours after a complete meal and 30 minutes to an hour following a light meal or snack. The amount of time depends largely upon what you have eaten, as certain types of food (carbohydrate, protein and fat) are digested at different rates. Generally, the higher the fat content, the slower the digestion rate. Protein also takes a bit longer to digest, while carbohydrates are digested more rapidly.

5. Drink at least 10 to 16 ounces (300 to 500 ml) of water before and after your sessions. You may also drink some water during your workout; however, if you pre-hydrate you can keep this to a minimum. Stopping to drink water too frequently reduces the effectiveness of your workout. Stay focused and keep moving. **Caution** – I am not advocating limiting water intake as some coaches have done in years past. This was done with the idea that they were developing discipline in their athletes. Although this was a common practice years ago, after a few athletes died from heat related illness, they decided it wasn't such a good idea after all.

Your body needs to be well hydrated in order to cool itself off. Drink plenty of water before you begin your session and stop for a drink only when you really need one, not as an excuse to rest. When you are is finished re-hydrate as needed.

6. Follow the plan as directed. Do not skip something or become lax when it comes to practicing visualization or logging your sessions. Each component of this program is vital to ensure the achievement of your goals.

Okay, by now you should have a good understanding of the process of goal setting and even set a few goals of your own. You also know the essential components of a balanced activity program and have a specific set of exercises to perform each day. The importance of keeping records has been explained, and you are equipped with sample recording forms on which to document your progress. Last but not least, you have been given some guidance with regard to your nutritional plan.

Now comes the all-important part of putting it all together to make the program work for you. I know for many of you these are major lifestyle changes I am asking you to make, changes that will not come easy at first. When you get discouraged, take some time to re-focus on your goals, and remember, anything of real value in life takes both time and effort. As you continue applying the principles taught in this program with both patience and persistence, you will experience miraculous changes in your life.

Your 24-Hour Guide to Optimal Health

Evening, before going to bed:

- Plan for the next day, including: wake-up time, activity session, meals and what you plan to accomplish at work, school, or around the house.

- Review your goals and practice visualization exercises.

- Sleep 7 to 8 hours or as needed for your body to recover.

The Next Morning:

- Wake-up as planned.

- Drink 10 to 16 ounces (300 to 500 ml) of water and eat a piece of fruit, small serving of starchy carbohydrate or something similar as your pre-workout snack. If fat loss is your goal you may want to exercise in a fasting state.

- Spend some quiet time in prayer and God's word. Review your goals and visualize yourself taking the necessary actions that will bring you closer to your dreams.

- Practice the exercises taught in the program for 10 to 30 minutes as your schedule allows with the rest of your day's activities.

- Replenish the water lost during your workout. If your session was particularly intense, eat a protein rich snack such as a protein shake or bar immediately following your workout to start the recovery process.

- Shower and get dressed.

- Enjoy a healthy breakfast beginning with:
  - Fresh fruit such as an orange, apple, banana, melon, or berries, depending on what may be in season.
  - A starchy carbohydrate source such as oatmeal, barley, whole grain bread, or sweet potato together with some nuts and seeds.
  - A source of omega fats that may come from your food or in the form of a supplement such as cod liver oil or fish oil capsules.

- Take a quality, whole food multi-vitamin/mineral supplement plus any other supplements that may be pertinent. Consult with your healthcare provider for additional guidance.

- Set your plan of action for the rest of your day into motion. With a good start to your day as outlined above, you will be energized and ready to go!

- Every hour or two take a few minutes to walk around, do some light stretching, breathing exercises or any movements to keep you energized?

Mid-morning:

- Eat a snack to maintain your energy level and boost your metabolism. A protein shake, energy bar, or nuts/seeds are good choices.

- Continue working for another 1 to 3 hours, depending on what you have scheduled before lunch. Drink a glass or two of water during this period to stay hydrated.

Afternoon:

- Time for a healthy lunch, consisting of:
  - A protein source such as lean meat, eggs, fish, or poultry.
  - A fibrous carbohydrate source: green and red peppers, leaf lettuce, broccoli, cabbage, kale or spinach are all good examples.

  Or if you prefer a carbohydrate rich meal:
  - A starchy carbohydrate source such as whole grain bread, brown rice, beans, sweet potatoes, or similar carbohydrate.

- A fibrous carbohydrate source: green and red peppers, leaf lettuce, broccoli, cabbage, kale or spinach are all good examples.

- Back to your *to do* list for the day. Time to stay focused on your goals and put energy toward the things that need to get done now. It is easy to put off less pleasant things for later, but if you really want to move forward in life, resist this temptation and do what you know needs to be done now!

- To avoid an afternoon lull, get up and do some light exercise to keep the blood flowing to your brain.

- Have a late afternoon snack now and/or following your activity session. Make sure to give yourself 30 to 90 minutes to digest before you begin to exercise.

- Get active for 10 to 30 minutes, depending on what you did in the morning and what you have scheduled for the rest of the evening.

- Enjoy a healthy dinner consisting of:
    - A protein source such as lean meat, eggs, fish, or poultry.

    - A fibrous carbohydrate source like green or red peppers, asparagus, broccoli, kale, spinach or any dark green leafy vegetables.

- Light exercise after your dinner may help you relax for a good night's sleep. Avoid any intense exercise late at night, as this will make it difficult to wind down and get to sleep.

- Review your day and plan for tomorrow as done the previous evening. Make sure to review your goals and practice visualization exercises.

Keep in mind, this is a **sample** day, a guide for you to use and then modify as needed to fit *your* day. It is important for you to establish a routine that works for you, one that you can stick with as you work toward the achievement of your goals.

As Stephen A. Brennan, an American Basketball Coach once said, "Our goals can only be reached through a vehicle of a plan, in which we must fervently believe, and upon which we must vigorously act. There is no other route to success."

I know that your efforts will bring you great success, and with each victory your confidence will soar, allowing you to reach beyond what you ever dreamed possible.

Coach David

You may contact me via email at: coachdavid@smartfittness.com

APPENDIX A

GOAL SETTING RECORDING FORM

<u>**Short-term Goals (1-2 months)**</u>

1. ____

   ____

   ____

   Action Plan:

   -

   -

   -

2. ____

   ____

   ____

   Action Plan:

   -

   -

   -

3. ____

   ____

   ____

   Action Plan:

   -

   -

   -

<u>**Intermediate Goals (3 – 6 months)**</u>

1. ____

____

____

Action Plan:

-

-

-

2. ____

____

____

Action Plan:

-

-

-

3. ____

____

____

Action Plan:

-

-

-

<u>**Long-term Goals (1 year)**</u>

1. ____

   ____

   ____

   Action Plan:

   -
   -
   -

2. ____

   ____

   ____

   Action Plan:

   -
   -
   -

3. ____

   ____

   ____

   Action Plan:

   -
   -
   -

<u>**Ultimate Long-term goals (3 – 5 years)**</u>

Here is your chance to dream a bit. Let your imagination go as you envision your life three to five years from now. Be prayerful as you consider God's will for your life and His plan for you.

____

____

____

____

____

____

____

____

____

____

____

____

____

____

____

____

____

APPENDIX B

A TO B WITH

A PURPOSE

RECORDING

FORM

A to B WITH A PURPOSE RECORDING FORM

DAY   DATE   ACTIVITY   TOTAL TIME   AVR HR *

______ ___/___/___ _____________ ___:___ ___bpm

______ ___/___/___ _____________ ___:___ ___bpm

______ ___/___/___ _____________ ___:___ ___bpm

______ ___/___/___ _____________ ___:___ ___bpm

______ ___/___/___ _____________ ___:___ ___bpm

______ ___/___/___ _____________ ___:___ ___bpm

______ ___/___/___ _____________ ___:___ ___bpm

______ ___/___/___ _____________ ___:___ ___bpm

______ ___/___/___ _____________ ___:___ ___bpm

______ ___/___/___ _____________ ___:___ ___bpm

*Heart rate data from your personal device such as a Polar heart rate monitor.

APPENDIX C
REAL-LIFE CONDITIONING RECORING FORM

<u>REAL-LIFE CONDITIONING RECORDING FORM</u>

Day ____________ Date ____/____/____ Time ____:____ Resting HR ______ bpm

Current State of Recovery: Recovered (At or below typical RHR) ____

Moderately Fatigued (5 bpm above RHR) ____ Fatigued (6 + bpm above RHR) ___

RHR = Resting Heart Rate   REPS = Repetitions   TUL = Time Under Load

<u>EXERCISE</u>	<u>REPS or TUL</u>	<u>NOTES</u>
__________	___/___/___	__________
__________	___/___/___	__________
__________	___/___/___	__________

Day ____________ Date ____/____/____ Time ____:____ Resting HR ______ bpm

__________	___/___/___	__________
__________	___/___/___	__________
__________	___/___/___	__________

Day ____________ Date ____/____/____ Time ____:____ Resting HR ______ bpm

__________	___/___/___	__________
__________	___/___/___	__________
__________	___/___/___	__________

Day ____________ Date ____/____/____ Time ____:____ Resting HR ______ bpm

__________	___/___/___	__________
__________	___/___/___	__________
__________	___/___/___	__________

www.ingramcontent.com/pod-product-compliance
Lightning Source LLC
Chambersburg PA
CBHW081723250726
48657CB00010B/3096